AN ADVANCED
ATLAS OF
Histology

By W. H. Freeman and Brian Bracegirdle

AN ATLAS OF EMBRYOLOGY
AN ATLAS OF HISTOLOGY
AN ADVANCED ATLAS OF HISTOLOGY
AN ATLAS OF INVERTEBRATE STRUCTURE

By Brian Bracegirdle and Patricia H. Miles

AN ATLAS OF PLANT STRUCTURE, Vol. 1
AN ATLAS OF PLANT STRUCTURE, Vol. 2
AN ATLAS OF CHORDATE STRUCTURE

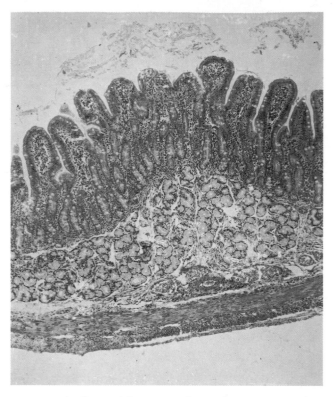

A. Stained haematoxylin and eosin

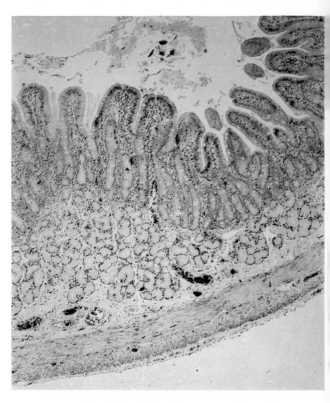

B. Stained iron haematoxylin

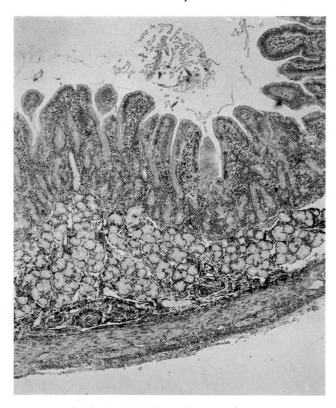

C. Stained Mallory-Azan trichrome

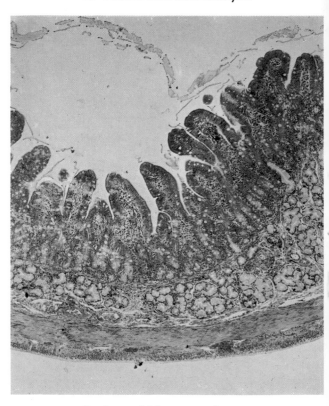

D. Stained Masson trichrome

RESULTS OF DIFFERENT STAINING TECHNIQUES

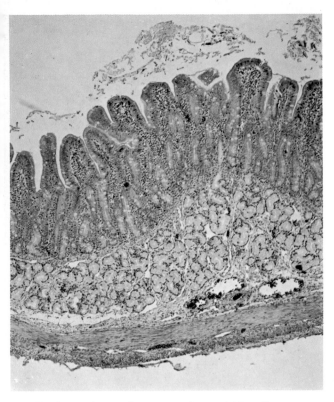

E. Stained iron haematoxylin and Van Gieson

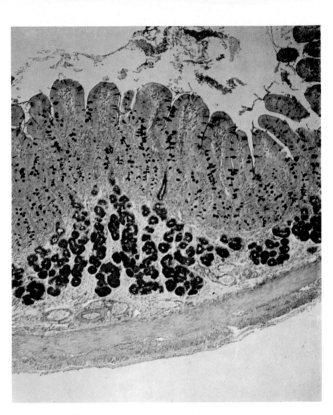

F. Stained P.A.S. and light green

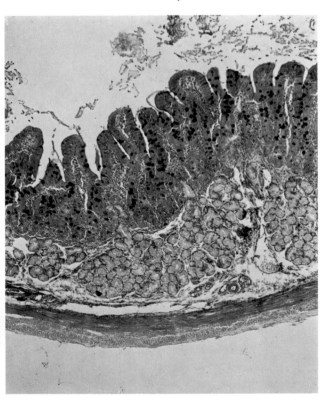

G. Stained Masson and aldehyde fuchsin

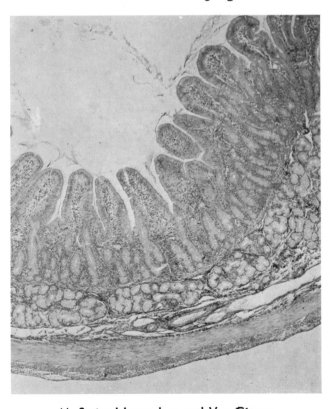

H. Stained haemalum and Van Gieson

DEMONSTRATED ON SECTIONS OF DUODENUM

AN ADVANCED
ATLAS OF
Histology

W H Freeman *BSc FIBiol*
formerly Head of Biology Department
Chislehurst and Sidcup Grammar School
formerly Chief Examiner 'A'-level Zoology, University of London

Brian Bracegirdle *BSc PhD FIBiol FRPS*

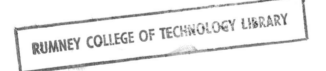
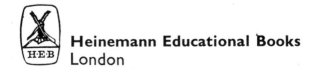
Heinemann Educational Books
London

Heinemann Educational Books Ltd.

22 Bedford Square, London WC1B 3HH

LONDON EDINBURGH MELBOURNE AUCKLAND
HONG KONG SINGAPORE KUALA LUMPUR NEW DELHI
IBADAN NAIROBI JOHANNESBURG
EXETER (NH) KINGSTON PORT OF SPAIN

ISBN 0 435 60317 5

© W. H. Freeman and Brian Bracegirdle 1976
First published 1976
Reprinted 1979, 1980

Colour plates printed by
George Over Ltd, Rugby

Printed at the University Press, Oxford
and bound in Great Britain by
Hunter & Foulis Ltd, Edinburgh

This Book is Dedicated to

DONALD CANWELL

Chief Technician of the Physiological Laboratory, Cambridge, mainstay of the supply of the preparations used in this book, and representative of that host of unsung technicians without whom work in histology would be totally impossible

Preface

This book, like all the others in the series, is designed for use at the laboratory bench, to guide the student in the interpretation of the structures seen with the microscope. Some summarised theoretical material has been included, but this Atlas is in no way intended to supplant one of the standard textbooks of histology which help the student equate structure with function.

All the photomicrographs and drawings have been specially made for the book, which contains material suitable for second medical degrees as well as reference material for work in school. We have been fortunate that preparations have been willingly lent for inclusion by histologists in many places. We must thank the following for their special help in this regard: Savile Bradbury, John Haller, John Kugler, Patricia Mitchell, David Turner, and especially Donald Canwell.

Our publishers have continued to be enthusiastic, and our families to be cheerful in the face of the many demands which the preparation of this book have placed on them.

W. H. F.
B. B.

January 1976

Colour Transparencies for Projection

Every photograph in this book is available as a 2×2 colour slide for projection from Philip Harris Biological Ltd., Oldmixon, Weston-super-Mare, Avon.

Each original master transparency was made at the same time as the negative for the corresponding picture in this book, exclusively for this Company. The authors recommend these slides for their quality and moderate cost as excellent aids to the teaching of histology especially in conjunction with this book.

CONTENTS

THE DIGESTIVE SYSTEM

THE SKIN

THE RESPIRATORY SYSTEM

THE NEUROSENSORY SYSTEM

THE ENDOCRINE SYSTEM

THE CIRCULATORY SYSTEM

THE LYMPHATIC SYSTEM

ORGAN RELATIONSHIPS

CELLS

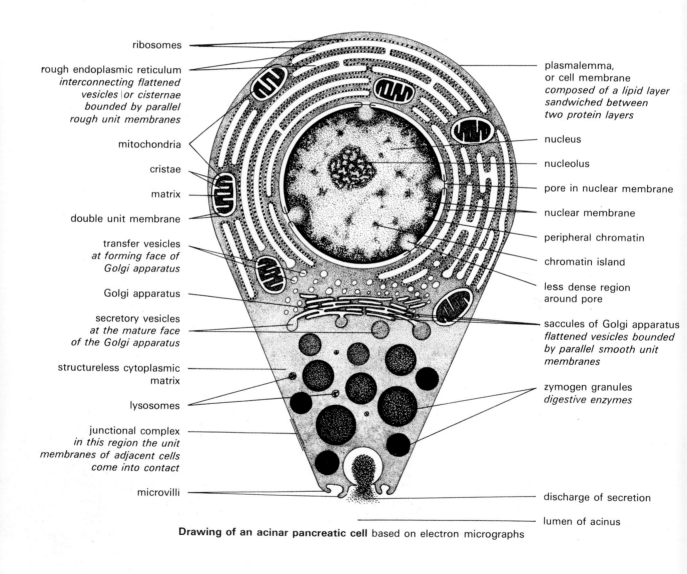

ribosomes

rough endoplasmic reticulum
*interconnecting flattened
vesicles | or cisternae
bounded by parallel
rough unit membranes*

mitochondria

cristae

matrix

double unit membrane

transfer vesicles
*at forming face of
Golgi apparatus*

Golgi apparatus

secretory vesicles
*at the mature face
of the Golgi apparatus*

structureless cytoplasmic
matrix

lysosomes

junctional complex
*in this region the unit
membranes of adjacent cells
come into contact*

microvilli

plasmalemma,
or cell membrane
*composed of a lipid layer
sandwiched between
two protein layers*

nucleus

nucleolus

pore in nuclear membrane

nuclear membrane

peripheral chromatin

chromatin island

less dense region
around pore

saccules of Golgi apparatus
*flattened vesicles bounded
by parallel smooth unit
membranes*

zymogen granules
digestive enzymes

discharge of secretion

lumen of acinus

Drawing of an acinar pancreatic cell based on electron micrographs

Cells are units of protoplasm surrounded by a plasma membrane. They vary in diameter from $7 \cdot 5\mu$ (erythrocytes of man) to 85 mm (ostrich egg). Usually each cell has a single nucleus separated from the cytoplasm by a perforated nuclear membrane: however, mammalian erythrocytes have no nuclei, while liver cells sometimes have two nuclei and osteoclasts seven or more. Cells are the functional units of the body capable of assimilating food, growing, respiring, excreting, secreting, responding to stimuli, and reproducing, though one or more of these functions may be lost in specialized cells. These activities depend upon cytoplasmic structures known as organelles.

The organelles of the cytoplasm are the endoplasmic reticulum, mitochondria, the Golgi apparatus, centrioles, ribosomes, and lysosomes. The structure of organelles can only be seen in electron micrographs. Non-living inclusions may occur in the cytoplasm — e.g. starch granules and fat droplets. Non-living material may also be produced outside cells — e.g. collagenous fibres and the matrix of bone.

The nuclei of cells stain darkly with haematoxylin and other basic dyes, whereas the cytoplasm stains with eosin, but there is no one staining technique which will demonstrate all cell components. The frontispiece shows the appearance of sections of duodenum stained by different techniques.

The chromosomes of a nucleus contain molecules of deoxyribonucleic acid (DNA) which carry coded information for the control of cytoplasmic functions. DNA molecules are far too large to be able to pass through the nuclear membrane and control the cytoplasm directly. Instead, sections of the coded information of DNA molecules are transcribed on to molecules of ribonucleic acid (RNA) which are much smaller and can pass through the nuclear membrane. It is by means of messenger RNA that the nucleus controls the cytoplasm.

With the exception of the gametes, every cell of an animal has the same number and kinds of chromosomes in its nucleus; in man the number of chromosomes is 46. Mitosis maintains this constancy by producing new nuclei with the same number and kinds of chromosomes as the parent nucleus. Before dividing the parent nucleus doubles its DNA content thereby ensuring that the new nuclei receive the same amounts of DNA as the parent nucleus as well as the same kinds. During mitosis the chromosomes coil and become stainable. Mitosis is a process of nuclear division; it is usually followed by cell division.

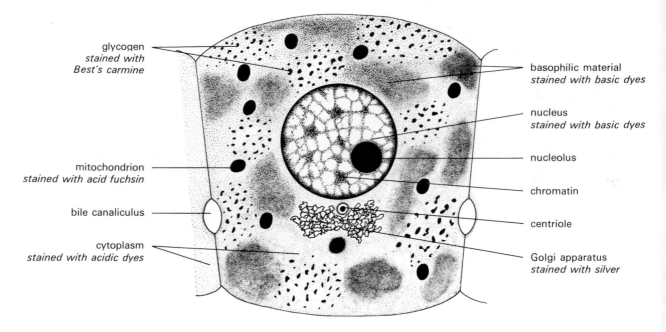

glycogen
*stained with
Best's carmine*

basophilic material
stained with basic dyes

nucleus
stained with basic dyes

nucleolus

mitochondrion
stained with acid fuchsin

chromatin

bile canaliculus

centriole

cytoplasm
stained with acidic dyes

Golgi apparatus
stained with silver

Diagram of a liver cell as seen with a light microscope.

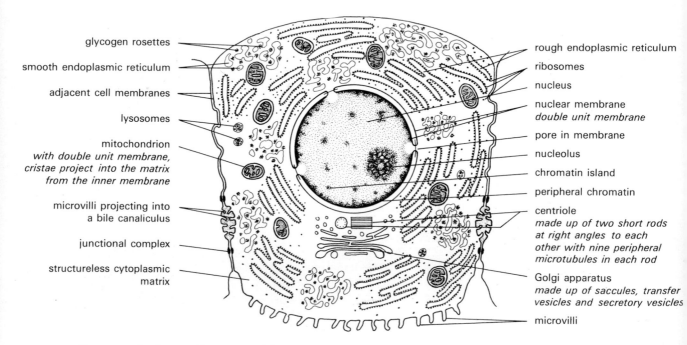

glycogen rosettes

smooth endoplasmic reticulum

adjacent cell membranes

lysosomes

mitochondrion
*with double unit membrane,
cristae project into the matrix
from the inner membrane*

microvilli projecting into
a bile canaliculus

junctional complex

structureless cytoplasmic
matrix

rough endoplasmic reticulum

ribosomes

nucleus

nuclear membrane
double unit membrane

pore in membrane

nucleolus

chromatin island

peripheral chromatin

centriole
*made up of two short rods
at right angles to each
other with nine peripheral
microtubules in each rod*

Golgi apparatus
*made up of saccules, transfer
vesicles and secretory vesicles*

microvilli

Diagram of a liver cell as seen with an electron microscope.

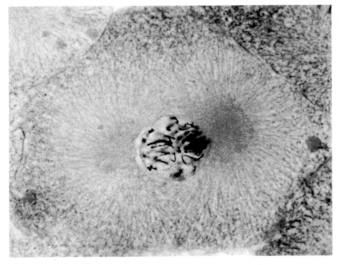

1. **Prophase** (whitefish blastula, T.S.), mag. 1100×

2. **Prometaphase** (whitefish blastula, T.S.), mag. 1100×

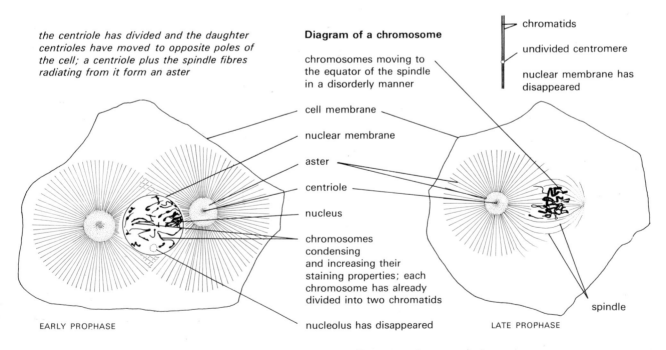

the centriole has divided and the daughter centrioles have moved to opposite poles of the cell; a centriole plus the spindle fibres radiating from it form an aster

Diagram of a chromosome

chromosomes moving to the equator of the spindle in a disorderly manner

chromatids

undivided centromere

nuclear membrane has disappeared

cell membrane

nuclear membrane

aster

centriole

nucleus

chromosomes condensing and increasing their staining properties; each chromosome has already divided into two chromatids

spindle

EARLY PROPHASE

LATE PROPHASE

nucleolus has disappeared

Drawing of specimen 1

Drawing of specimen 2

3

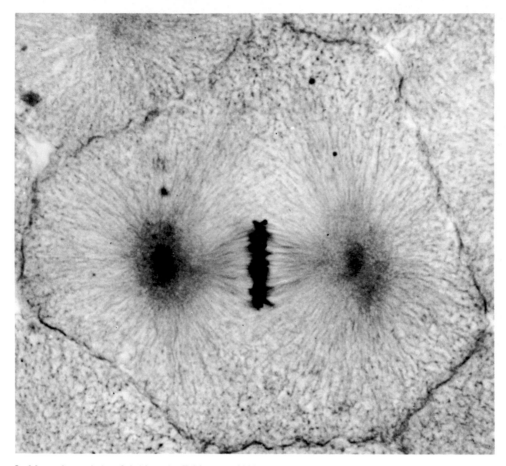

3. **Metaphase** (whitefish blastula, T.S.), mag. 1100 ×

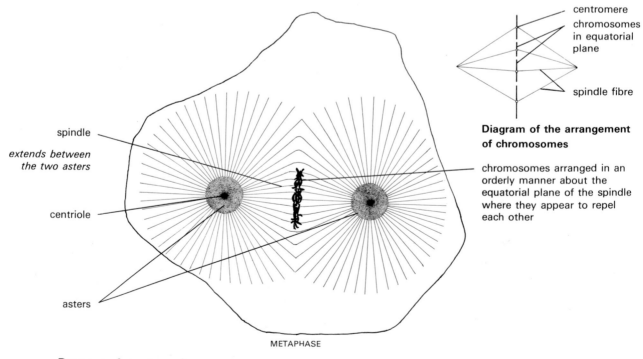

centromere

chromosomes in equatorial plane

spindle fibre

Diagram of the arrangement of chromosomes

spindle

extends between the two asters

centriole

asters

chromosomes arranged in an orderly manner about the equatorial plane of the spindle where they appear to repel each other

METAPHASE

Drawing of specimen 3

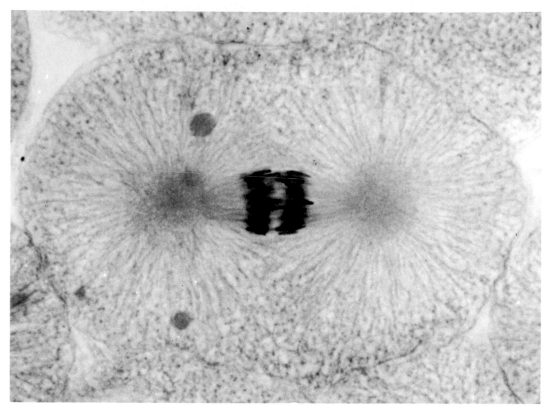

4. **Anaphase** (whitefish blastula, T.S.), mag. 1100×

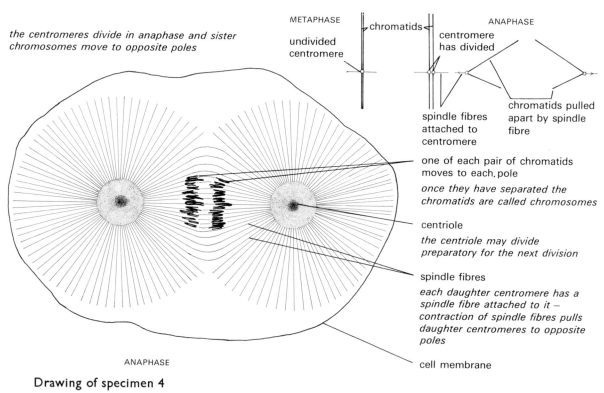

the centromeres divide in anaphase and sister chromosomes move to opposite poles

METAPHASE

chromatids

undivided centromere

spindle fibres attached to centromere

ANAPHASE

centromere has divided

chromatids pulled apart by spindle fibre

one of each pair of chromatids moves to each pole

once they have separated the chromatids are called chromosomes

centriole

the centriole may divide preparatory for the next division

spindle fibres

each daughter centromere has a spindle fibre attached to it – contraction of spindle fibres pulls daughter centromeres to opposite poles

ANAPHASE

cell membrane

Drawing of specimen 4

5

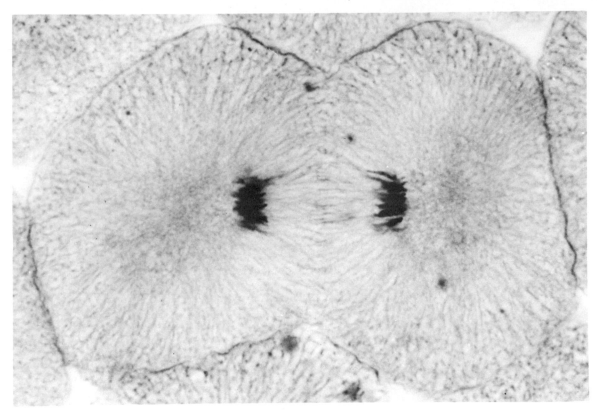

5. **Telophase** (whitefish blastula, T.S.), mag. 1100×

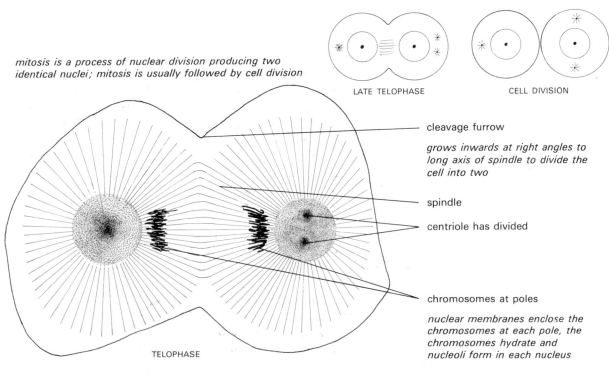

*mitosis is a process of nuclear division producing two
identical nuclei; mitosis is usually followed by cell division*

LATE TELOPHASE

CELL DIVISION

cleavage furrow

*grows inwards at right angles to
long axis of spindle to divide the
cell into two*

spindle

centriole has divided

chromosomes at poles

*nuclear membranes enclose the
chromosomes at each pole, the
chromosomes hydrate and
nucleoli form in each nucleus*

TELOPHASE

Drawing of specimen 5

TISSUES

A fertilized egg divides to form several smaller cells which are very much alike. After they have undergone morphogenetic movements, these cells become arranged in three germ layers, the ectoderm, endoderm, and mesoderm. The cells of each layer then differentiate along divergent lines to produce the tissues of the body.

A simple tissue may be defined as a group of cells of common origin having the same specialized structure which fits them to perform a common function. Such a simple tissue is, however, uncommon apart from epithelia, and most tissues are complex, being made up of several different kinds of cells. Tissues are the building blocks that form the organs. A sound knowledge of the tissues is therefore essential before an attempt can be made to study the structure of organs.

There are four categories of tissue:

epithelial tissue – derived from all three germ layers
connective tissue – derived from mesoderm
muscular tissue – derived from mesoderm
nervous tissue – derived from ectoderm.

EPITHELIAL TISSUE

There are two types of epithelia: A – covering epithelia, and B – glandular epithelia.

A. COVERING EPITHELIA

1. The cells form a continuous layer covering an internal or external surface.

2. The cells are held together at their common boundaries by a thin layer of intercellular substance.

3. One surface of each cell is free and often highly specialized.

4. The opposite surface rests on a basement membrane derived from the underlying connective tissue.

5. Blood vessels are absent.

6. Covering epithelia are exposed to physical injury and infection and act as protective layers.

7. Damaged cells are replaced by new ones and mitotic figures are common.

8. All the vital traffic of the body passes through epithelia – e.g. digested food, oxygen, waste products, secretions.

9. Some epithelia are specialized for the reception of stimuli.

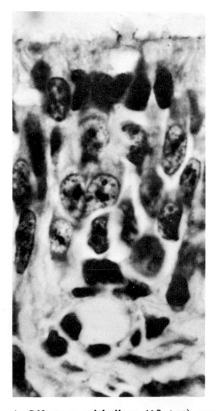

6. **Olfactory epithelium,** V.S. (cat), mag. 1400×

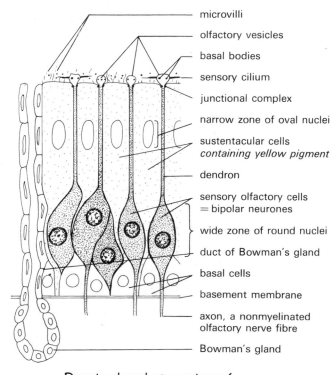

microvilli
olfactory vesicles
basal bodies
sensory cilium
junctional complex
narrow zone of oval nuclei
sustentacular cells
containing yellow pigment
dendron
sensory olfactory cells
= bipolar neurones
wide zone of round nuclei
duct of Bowman's gland
basal cells
basement membrane
axon, a nonmyelinated
olfactory nerve fibre
Bowman's gland

Drawing based on specimen 6

Classification of Covering Epithelia

Covering epithelia are classified according to either the arrangement or the shape of the constituent cells.

CLASSIFICATION BASED ON CELL ARRANGEMENT

1. Simple epithelia – these are one cell thick.

2. Pseudostratified epithelia – these appear to be more than one cell thick but all the cells rest on the basement membrane.

3. Stratified epithelia – these are many cells thick.

CLASSIFICATION BASED ON CELL SHAPES

1. Squamous epithelia – these are made up of flattened cells shaped like paving stones.

2. Cuboidal epithelia – are made of isodiametric cells.

3. Columnar epithelia – consist of cells which are taller than they are wide.

4. Transitional epithelia – these are made up of cells which change their shape when the epithelium is stretched.

There are twelve possible classes if these two schemes of classification are combined, but only eight of these occur.

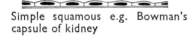
Simple squamous e.g. Bowman's capsule of kidney

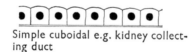
Simple cuboidal e.g. kidney collecting duct

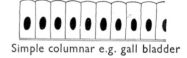
Simple columnar e.g. gall bladder

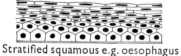
Stratified squamous e.g. oesophagus

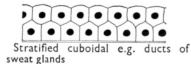
Stratified cuboidal e.g. ducts of sweat glands

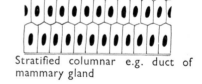
Stratified columnar e.g. duct of mammary gland

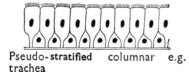
Pseudo-stratified columnar e.g. trachea

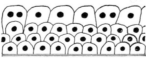

a) relaxed   Stratified transitional e.g. bladder

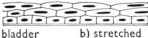
b) stretched

CLASSES OF COVERING EPITHELIA

B. GLANDULAR EPITHELIA

All living cells secrete and some, such as goblet cells, are highly specialized for this purpose. A gland is an organ largely composed of specialized secretory cells. The material secreted is usually a liquid containing such substances as enzymes, hormones, mucin, or fats.

Glands are epithelial in origin. The epithelial nature of the mucous membrane of the stomach is obvious. In most cases, however, the elaborate folding and branching of the invaginated epithelial layer that occur during development obscure the epithelial nature of glands.

Exocrine glands remain connected to a surface epithelium by the ducts through which they discharge their secretions. Endocrine glands, on the other hand, have no ducts and lose their epithelial connections. These ductless glands are highly vascular and discharge their secretions into blood vessels.

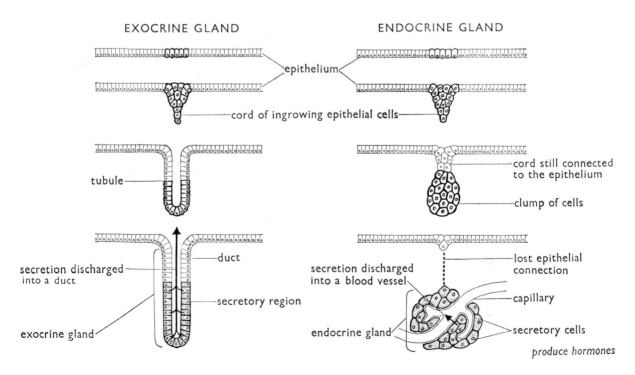

EXOCRINE GLAND   ENDOCRINE GLAND

epithelium

cord of ingrowing epithelial cells

tubule

cord still connected to the epithelium

clump of cells

secretion discharged into a duct

duct

secretory region

exocrine gland

secretion discharged into a blood vessel

lost epithelial connection

capillary

secretory cells

endocrine gland

produce hormones

DIAGRAM TO SHOW THE EPITHELIAL ORIGIN OF GLANDS

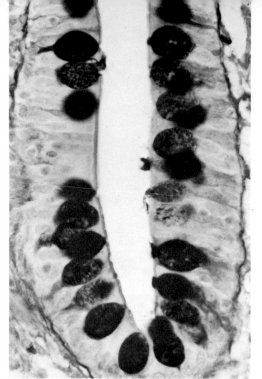

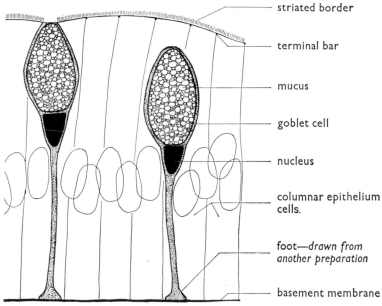

striated border

terminal bar

mucus

goblet cell

nucleus

columnar epithelium cells.

foot—*drawn from another preparation*

basement membrane

7. **Goblet cells** (mammalian ileum, V.S.), mag. 950×

Drawing based on specimen 7

Secretions are produced by three distinct methods:

1. Merocrine. The secretion accumulates below the free surface of the cell through which it is released. There is no loss of cytoplasm. Merocrine secretion is exhibited by goblet cells and sweat glands.

2. Apocrine. The secretion accumulates below the free surface but can only be released by the breaking away of the distal part of the cell thus involving cytoplasmic loss. The mammary glands secrete milk in this manner.

3. Holocrine. The secretion is formed by the complete break-down of the secretory cells. Sebaceous glands are holocrine.

The ovary and testis are sometimes described as being cytogenous glands whose secretions are the germ cells.

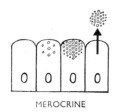

MEROCRINE

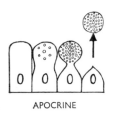

APOCRINE

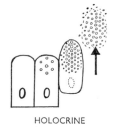

HOLOCRINE

DIAGRAM ILLUSTRATING SECRETION

Classification of Exocrine Glands

Glands are classified according to the shape of the secretory part (tubular or alveolar), and the nature of the ducts. If the duct is unbranched the gland is said to be simple; compound glands have branched ducts.

    1. *Simple tubular*, e.g. crypt of Lieberkühn.

    2. *Simple coiled tubular*, e.g. sweat gland.

    3. *Simple branched tubular*, e.g. fundic gland (only the secretory part is branched).

    4. *Simple alveolar*, e.g. mucous and poison glands in skin of frog (the term saccular is sometimes used for alveolar glands with a large lumen).

    5. *Simple branched alveolar*, e.g. Meibomian gland (only the secretory part is branched).

    6. *Compound tubular*, e.g. gland of Brunner (this is sometimes classified as a tubulo-alveolar gland since some secretory units are dilated).

    7. *Compound alveolar*, e.g. lactating mammary gland.

    8. *Compound tubulo-alveolar*, e.g. submaxillary gland.

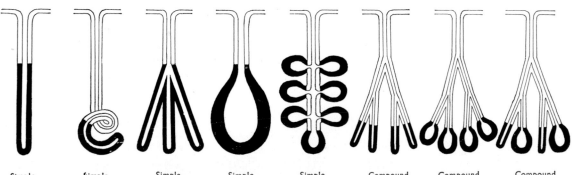

| Simple tubular | Simple coiled tubular | Simple branched tubular | Simple alveolar | Simple branched alveolar | Compound tubular | Compound alveolar | Compound tubulo-alveolar |

DIAGRAM TO ILLUSTRATE THE VARIOUS TYPES OF GLAND

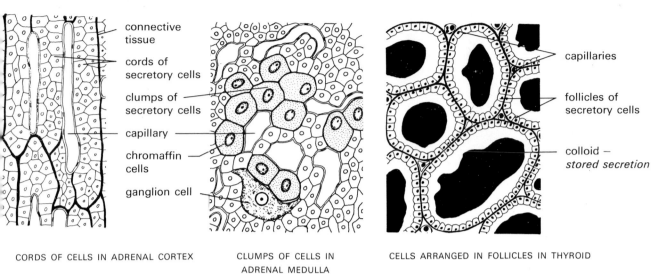

connective tissue	
cords of secretory cells	
clumps of secretory cells	
capillary	
chromaffin cells	
ganglion cell	

capillaries

follicles of secretory cells

colloid – *stored secretion*

CORDS OF CELLS IN ADRENAL CORTEX   CLUMPS OF CELLS IN ADRENAL MEDULLA   CELLS ARRANGED IN FOLLICLES IN THYROID

Diagram to illustrate the various types of endocrine gland.

Endocrine glands

Endocrine glands are organs whose function is to secrete hormones, e.g. the pituitary (see pp. 134, 135), the adrenal (see pp. 137, 138, 139), the thyroid (see p. 136), and the parathyroid (see pp. 134, 135).

Several other organs secrete hormones in addition to performing their main functions, e.g. stomach wall, duodenal wall, kidney cortex – the juxtaglomerular cells of which secrete renin, pancreas (see pp. 80, 81) and gonads (see pp. 90, 91, 97, 98, 99, 103).

Hormones act on targets some distance away from endocrine tissues; they are transported to their targets by the blood vascular system. This dependence on the blood system is reflected in the arrangement of secretory cells in cords or clumps. The secretory cells of the adrenal cortex are a good example of the cord type of arrangement in which columns of cells are separated from each other by capillaries. The chromaffin cells of the adrenal medulla occur in clumps, each clump being surrounded by a network of capillaries. Both these arrangements facilitate the discharge of hormones into blood vessels.

Secretory products, instead of being discharged as they are formed, are stored within endocrine glands. In most cases this is done by intracellular storage but there is a limit to the amount of secretion that can be retained within cells. Some form of extracellular storage is necessary for the accumulation of large amounts of secretion.

The follicles of the thyroid gland are spherical or sausage-shaped bags whose walls consist of a single layer of cuboidal cells. These cells discharge their secretion into the cavity of a follicle where it can be stored until required.

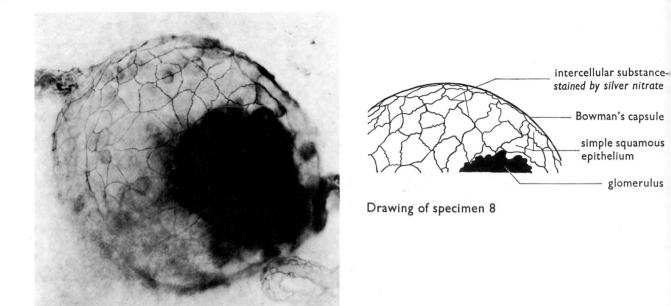

intercellular substance-
stained by silver nitrate

Bowman's capsule

simple squamous
epithelium

glomerulus

Drawing of specimen 8

8. **Simple squamous epithelium,** E. (mammalian kidney, T.S.), mag. 350×

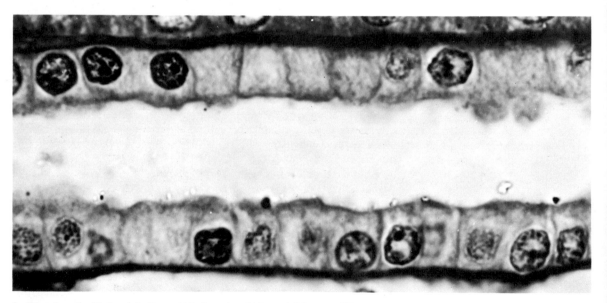

9. **Simple cuboidal epithelium,** V.S. (monkey kidney, L.S.), mag. 800×

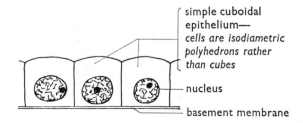

simple cuboidal
epithelium—
*cells are isodiametric
polyhedrons rather
than cubes*

nucleus

basement membrane

Drawing based on specimen 9 (idealised and simplified)

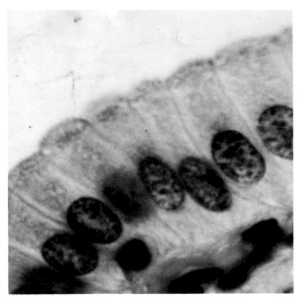

10. Simple columnar epithelium, V.S.
(human gall bladder, T.S.), mag. 1150×

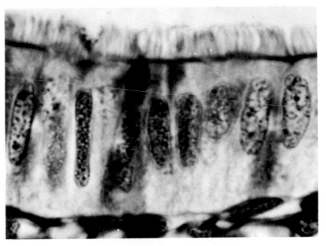

11. Simple ciliated columnar epithelium, V.S.
(rabbit oviduct, T.S.), mag. 1150×

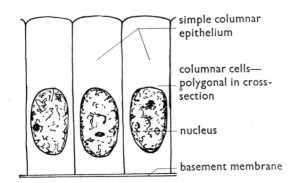

simple columnar epithelium

columnar cells—polygonal in cross-section

nucleus

basement membrane

Drawing based on specimen 10 (idealised and simplified)

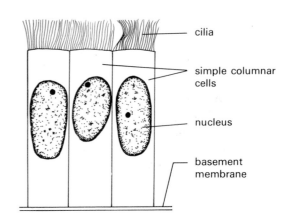

cilia

simple columnar cells

nucleus

basement membrane

Drawing based on specimen 11 (idealised and simplified)

15

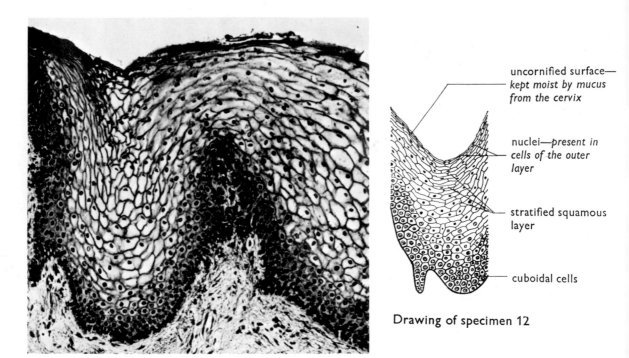

uncornified surface—
kept moist by mucus
from the cervix

nuclei—present in
cells of the outer
layer

stratified squamous
layer

cuboidal cells

Drawing of specimen 12

12. **Stratified squamous epithelium,** V.S. (human vagina, L.S.), mag. 200×

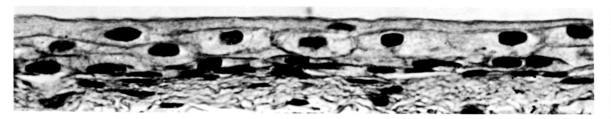

13. **Transitional epithelium,** stretched, V.S. (monkey bladder, T.S.), mag. 250×

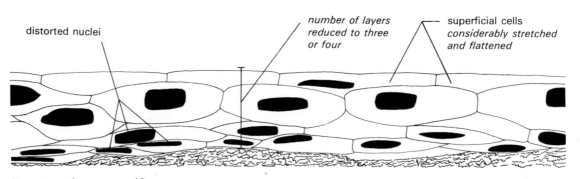

distorted nuclei

*number of layers
reduced to three
or four*

*superficial cells
considerably stretched
and flattened*

Drawing of specimen 13

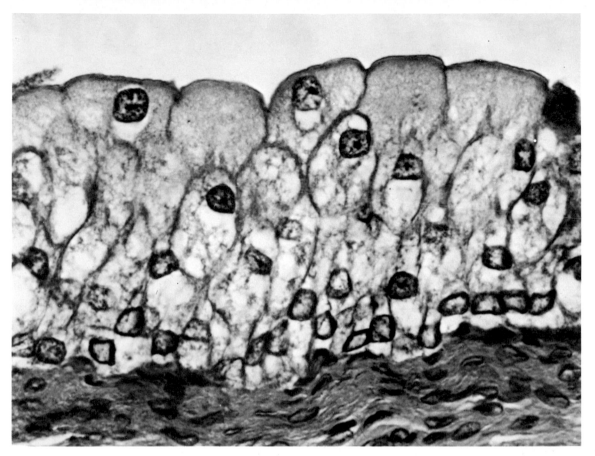

14. **Transitional epithelium,** relaxed, V.S. (rat bladder, T.S.), mag. 125×

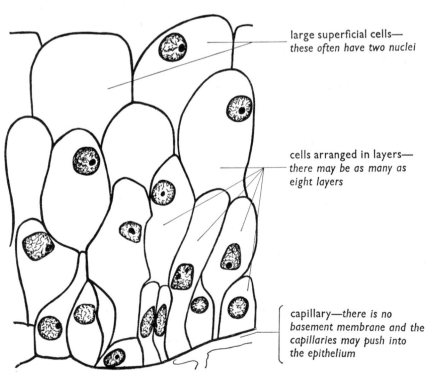

large superficial cells—
these often have two nuclei

cells arranged in layers—
*there may be as many as
eight layers*

capillary—*there is no
basement membrane and the
capillaries may push into
the epithelium*

Drawing of specimen 14

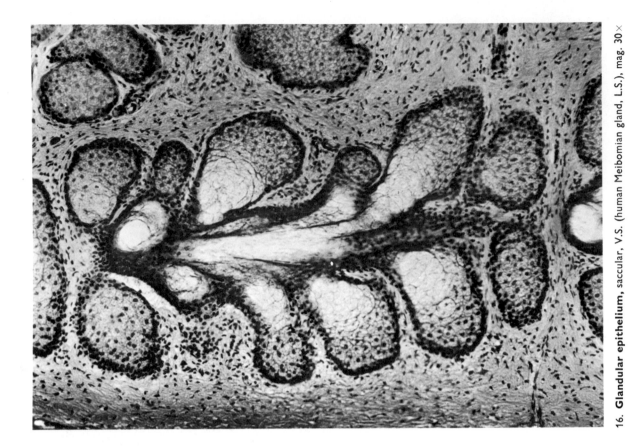

16. **Glandular epithelium,** saccular, V.S. (human Meibomian gland, L.S.), mag. 30×

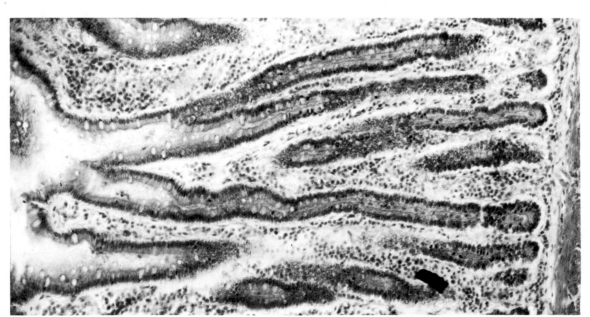

15. **Glandular epithelium,** simple tubular, V.S. (human ileum, L.S.), mag. 85×

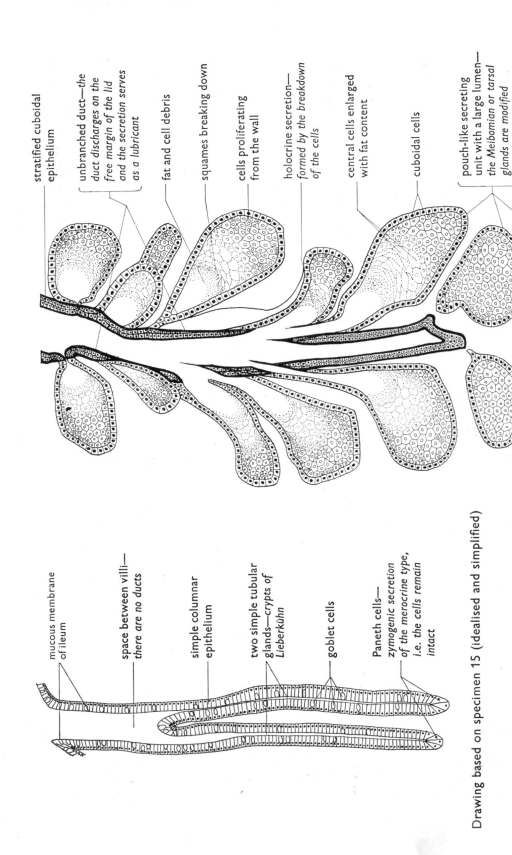

stratified cuboidal epithelium

unbranched duct—*the duct discharges on the free margin of the lid and the secretion serves as a lubricant*

fat and cell debris

squames breaking down

cells proliferating from the wall

holocrine secretion—*formed by the breakdown of the cells*

central cells enlarged with fat content

cuboidal cells

pouch-like secreting unit with a large lumen—*the Meibomian or tarsal glands are modified sebaceous glands*

Drawing based on specimen 16 (the drawing is of an adjacent section in a series)

mucous membrane of ileum

space between villi—*there are no ducts*

simple columnar epithelium

two simple tubular glands—*crypts of Lieberkühn*

goblet cells

Paneth cells—*zymogenic secretion of the merocrine type, i.e. the cells remain intact*

Drawing based on specimen 15 (idealised and simplified)

CONNECTIVE TISSUE

Early in the process of development stellate mesenchyme cells break away from the mesoderm, and these wandering cells become distributed between the three germ layers throughout the embryo. Connective tissue arises from these widely scattered free mesenchyme cells and is correspondingly ubiquitous in its distribution. Some of the mesenchyme cells remain in an undifferentiated condition in adult tissue.

Connective tissue is made up of cells, ground substance or matrix, and fibres. Matrix and fibres, which are non-living products of the cells, predominate, and form the supporting material of the body. As the name suggests, connective tissue serves as a connecting system binding all other tissues together.

Connective tissue forms sheaths around organs, bundles in which lie nerves and blood vessels, and sheets or fascia attaching the skin to underlying tissues.

The art of dissection is to display organs by separating them from their envelopes of obscuring connective tissue.

The sheaths around organs separate them from one another, enabling each organ to perform its special functions without interference from neighbouring organs. They also serve in defence against bacterial invasion, inflammation being an indication that a particular region has been invaded. Fat is stored in the superficial fascia, and this layer of adipose tissue provides insulation against heat losses from the skin. The skeletal framework of the body depends upon the specialized matrices of bone and cartilage for its rigidity.

Yet another kind of connective tissue, the haemopoietic tissue, is responsible for the production of blood cells.

The factor common to these diverse tissues is their origin from mesenchyme cells.

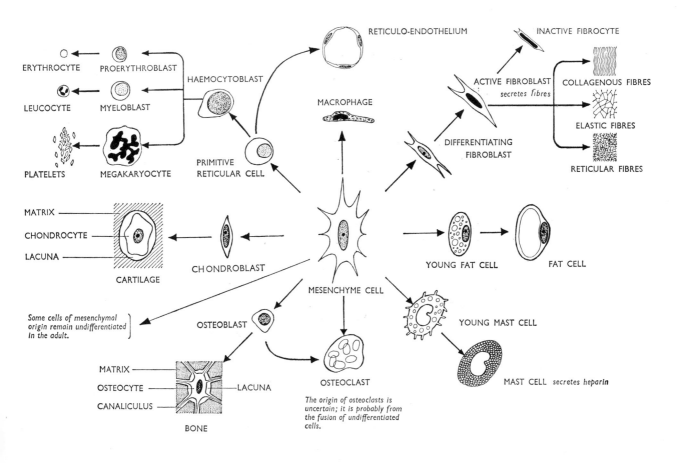

ERYTHROCYTE
PROERYTHROBLAST
HAEMOCYTOBLAST
RETICULO-ENDOTHELIUM
INACTIVE FIBROCYTE

LEUCOCYTE
MYELOBLAST
MACROPHAGE
ACTIVE FIBROBLAST *secretes fibres*
COLLAGENOUS FIBRES

PLATELETS
MEGAKARYOCYTE
PRIMITIVE RETICULAR CELL
DIFFERENTIATING FIBROBLAST
ELASTIC FIBRES

RETICULAR FIBRES

MATRIX
CHONDROCYTE
LACUNA
CHONDROBLAST
YOUNG FAT CELL
FAT CELL

CARTILAGE

Some cells of mesenchymal origin remain undifferentiated in the adult.

MESENCHYME CELL

OSTEOBLAST
YOUNG MAST CELL

MATRIX
OSTEOCYTE
CANALICULUS
LACUNA
OSTEOCLAST
MAST CELL *secretes heparin*

BONE

The origin of osteoclasts is uncertain; it is probably from the fusion of undifferentiated cells.

DIAGRAM ILLUSTRATING THE MAIN TYPES OF CONNECTIVE TISSUE CELLS
DERIVED FROM EMBRYONIC MESENCHYME

Shrinkage

Fixation is the first stage in the preparation of fresh material for examination under a microscope. A certain amount of distortion occurs in all fixatives and if the process is done badly the tissues shrink so much that spaces develop between them.

Connective tissue, because of its mixed composition of cells, fibres and matrix, is particularly susceptible to shrinkage.

Classification of Connective Tissues

Connective tissues are classified according to the nature and arrangement of their non-living components. The classification below is based on that of Ham.

1. *Loose or areolar tissue.* A jelly-like ground substance containing cells and a loose network of fibres, e.g. in subcutaneous connective tissue.

2. *Adipose.* Similar to areolar tissue, but cells storing fat predominate, e.g. fat depots round the kidney.

3. *Dense fibrous.* Fibres predominate: a. regularly arranged, e.g. tendon, ligament, elastic ligament; b. irregularly arranged, e.g. dermis.

4. *Reticular.* A network of fine branching reticular fibres, which stain with silver, supporting parenchymal cells of viscera, e.g. spleen, liver.

5. *Cartilage.* A firm plastic matrix, containing fibres: a. Hyaline – translucent matrix with very fine collagen fibres, e.g. cartilage of trachea; b. Fibro-cartilage – dense collagenous fibres embedded in matrix, e.g. intervertebral disc; c. Elastic cartilage – elastic fibres embedded in matrix, e.g. cartilage of pinna, epiglottis.

6. *Bone.* Solid rigid matrix, containing collagenous fibres:
a. Spongy bone – trabeculae of bone between marrow-containing cavities, e.g. epiphysis of long bones, and inner regions of flat bones; b. Dense bone – formed of Haversian systems (osteones), e.g. shaft of long bones.

7. *Dentine.* Matrix similar to bone, e.g. teeth.

8. *Haemopoietic.* a. Myeloid, e.g. red marrow of ribs; b. Lymphatic, e.g. spleen, lymph nodes.

INTERCELLULAR SUBSTANCE

The following types of intercellular substance occur in connective tissue:

1. *amorphous ground substance*
2. *fibres: collagenous, elastic, reticular*
3. *matrix of cartilage, bone, dentine.*

Connective tissue cells depend on the diffusion of nutrient and waste materials in minute channels in bone and dentine, and through the amorphous matrix of all other connective tissues. Tissue fluid, an exudate of blood plasma, provides the medium for diffusion. An abnormal accumulation of this fluid occurs if its drainage into the lymphatic capillaries is impeded, resulting in the condition called oedema.

1. *Amorphous ground substance.* Composed of a mixture of mucopolysaccharides, e.g. hyaluronic acid and chondroitin sulphate with other unidentified substances.

Some bacteria invade connective tissue by secreting an enzyme, hyaluronidase, which digests the hyaluronic acid of the ground substance.

The amorphous material is metachromatic (i.e. it stains characteristically with toluidine blue and thionine, changing the colour of the stain), and gives a positive periodic acid Schiff reaction (i.e. carbohydrates present are oxidised by periodic acid to give aldehyde groups visualized with Schiff's reagent).

Basement membranes of epithelia are chemically similar to amorphous ground substance, and are PAS positive.

2. *Fibres.* Fibroblasts are connective tissue cells that secrete a fibre precursor which is condensed to collagen either within the cell or, more probably, on the cell surface. Fibroblasts are also thought to be responsible for the synthesis of elastic and reticular fibres and for the amorphous components of the intercellular substance.

TABLE SUMMARISING THE PROPERTIES OF FIBRES

	COLLAGEN	ELASTIC	RETICULAR
appearance	colourless–hence known as white fibres	yellow – hence known as yellow fibres	only demonstrated by special silver techniques – hence called argyrophilic fibres
distribution	wide, particularly in tendon, joint capsules and ligaments	blood vessels, particularly aorta, lung, elastic ligaments, vocal cords	lymphatic system, particularly spleen; support basement membranes
structure	coarse; long fibres in wavy bundles; no branching; fibrils present	fine fibres which branch to form a network; no fibrils	fine short fibres which branch to form a close network; a few fibrils present
striations	electron micrographs reveal transverse striations, periodicity 640 A or 2,600 A	none	striations with periodicity of those of collagen fibres
tensile strength	great	little	little
elasticity	flexible but inelastic	considerable	little
refractive index	low	high	low
chemical composition	collagen, yields glycine on hydrolysis; boiling yields gelatin	elastin, yielding glycine and leucine on hydrolysis	reticulin, similar to collagen but exact nature unknown
pepsin digestion	rapid	resistant	
trypsin digestion	none	slow	none
weak acids and alkalis	cause swelling; dissolve	resistant	resistant
staining reactions:			
van Gieson	red	yellow	—
H. and E	pink	—	—
Mallory	blue	—	blue
Masson	green	—	green
resorcin fuchsin	—	dark purple	—
orcein	—	dark brown	—
silver	brown with some techniques	—	black

3. *Matrix*. The matrix of cartilage is composed of three substances:
   a. Chondromucoid – a glycoprotein
   b. Chrondroitin sulphate – strongly basophilic
   c. Albumoid – amount present increases with age.

The amorphous substance is permeated by fine collagenous fibres which are not visible in routine preparations.

The matrix of bone consists of a mineral component (about 65 per cent) and an organic component. The mineral matter is a compound of calcium and phosphate having the structure of a hydroxyapatite, $3Ca_3(PO_4)_2.Ca(OH)_2$. Some calcium carbonate is also present.

The organic matter is ossein which is very similar to collagen, yielding gelatin on boiling.

Dentine contains 70 per cent mineral matter and is similar to bone but harder. It is formed by odontoblasts; these cells send out slender processes which lie in the dentinal canals.

Transitional regions

Where two different types of connective tissue meet there is a transitional region at the junction where one type merges into the other, e.g. the insertion of tendons at a bony or cartilagenous surface.

Metaplasia

One type of connective tissue sometimes gives rise to another type, e.g. the pathological formation of nodules of bone in tendons. This is not due to conversion of tendon to bone. These metaplasia occur because the undifferentiated mesenchyme cells produce bone instead of tendon.

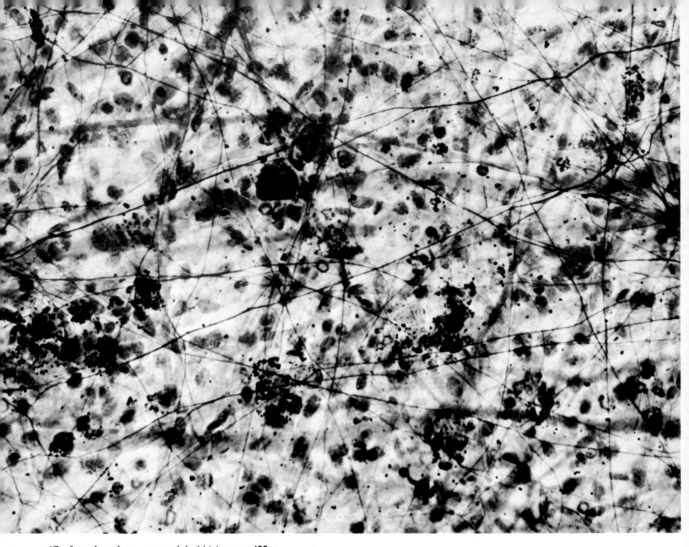

17. **Areolar tissue**, spread (rabbit), mag. 400×

18. **Tendon**, L.S. (human), mag. 350×

19. **Adipose tissue**, T.S. (cat), mag. 375×

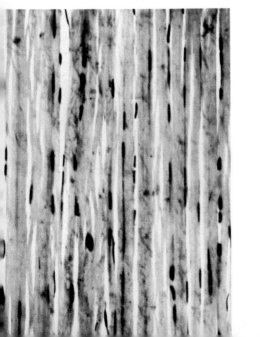

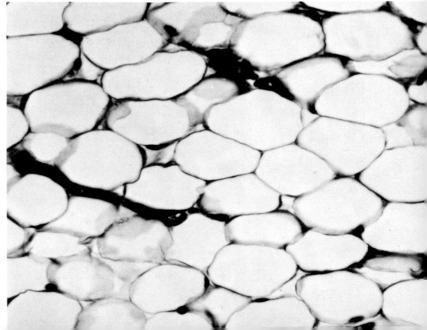

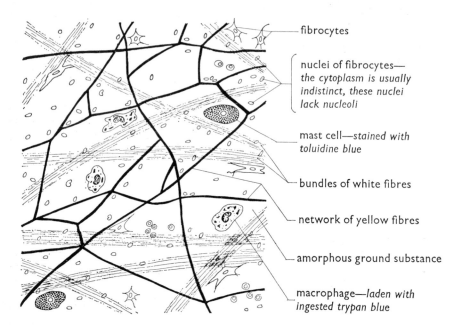

— fibrocytes

nuclei of fibrocytes—
*the cytoplasm is usually
indistinct, these nuclei
lack nucleoli*

mast cell—*stained with
toluidine blue*

bundles of white fibres

network of yellow fibres

amorphous ground substance

macrophage—*laden with
ingested trypan blue*

Drawing based on specimen 17

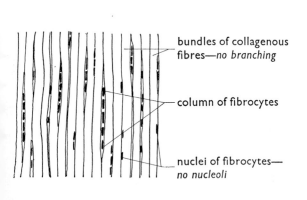

bundles of collagenous
fibres—*no branching*

column of fibrocytes

nuclei of fibrocytes—
no nucleoli

Drawing of specimen 18

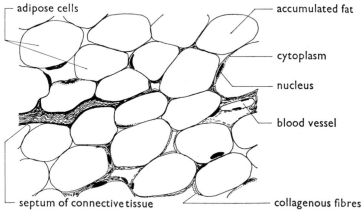

adipose cells

accumulated fat

cytoplasm

nucleus

blood vessel

septum of connective tissue

collagenous fibres

Drawing of specimen 19

Note
Fat is soluble in many of the solvents
used in the preparation of material.
Adipose cells, as a consequence, are
usually empty in prepared slides.

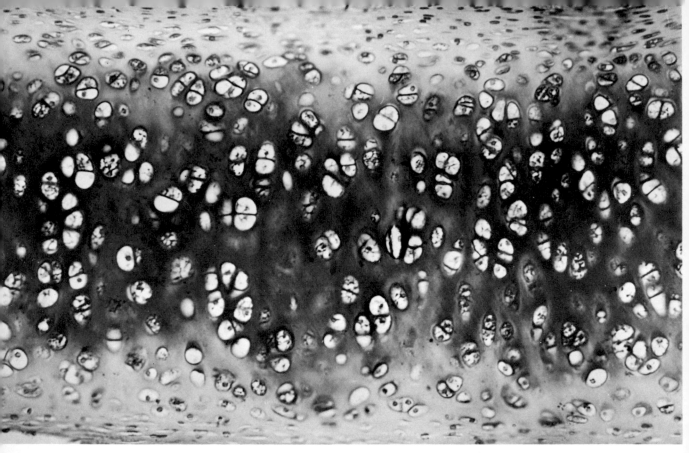

20. **Hyaline cartilage,** T.S. (human trachea, T.S.), mag. 200 ×

21. **White fibrous cartilage,** L.S.
(baboon patellar tendon insertion, L.S.), mag. 120 ×

22. **Yellow elastic cartilage,** V.S
(human pinna, T.S.), mag. 75 ×

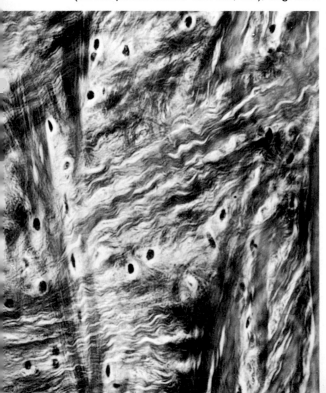

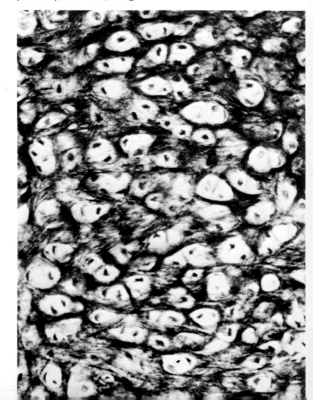

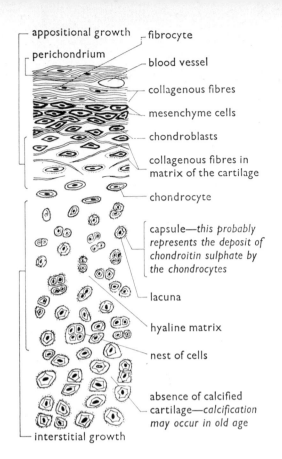

- appositional growth
- perichondrium
- fibrocyte
- blood vessel
- collagenous fibres
- mesenchyme cells
- chondroblasts
- collagenous fibres in matrix of the cartilage
- chondrocyte
- capsule—*this probably represents the deposit of chondroitin sulphate by the chondrocytes*
- lacuna
- hyaline matrix
- nest of cells
- absence of calcified cartilage—*calcification may occur in old age*
- interstitial growth

Diagram to explain specimen 20

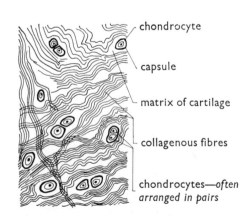

- chondrocyte
- capsule
- matrix of cartilage
- collagenous fibres
- chondrocytes—*often arranged in pairs*

Drawing based on specimen 21
(idealised and simplified)

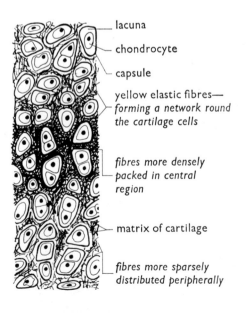

- lacuna
- chondrocyte
- capsule
- yellow elastic fibres—*forming a network round the cartilage cells*
- *fibres more densely packed in central region*
- matrix of cartilage
- *fibres more sparsely distributed peripherally*

Drawing of specimen 22

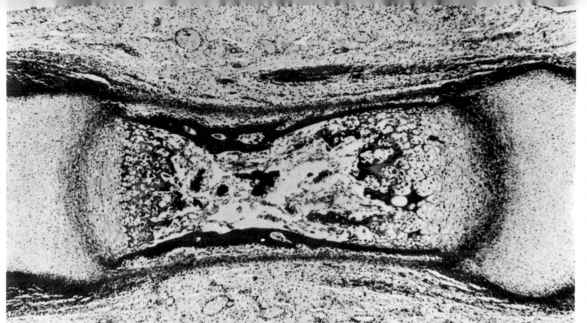

24. **Ossification,** perichondral and endochondral, L.S. (human foetal phalanx, L.S.), mag. 30 ×

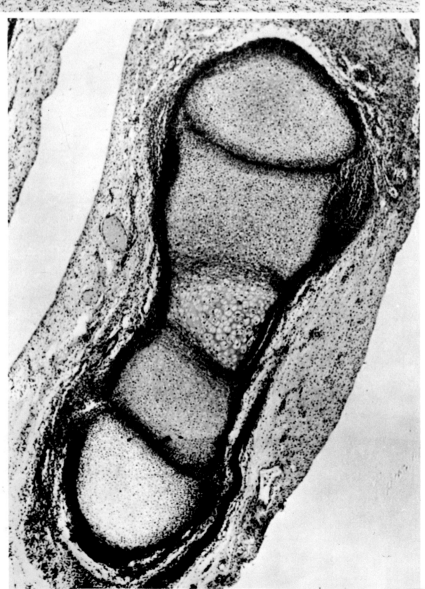

23. **Ossification,** cartilage model, L.S. (human foetal phalanx, L.S.) mag. 30 ×

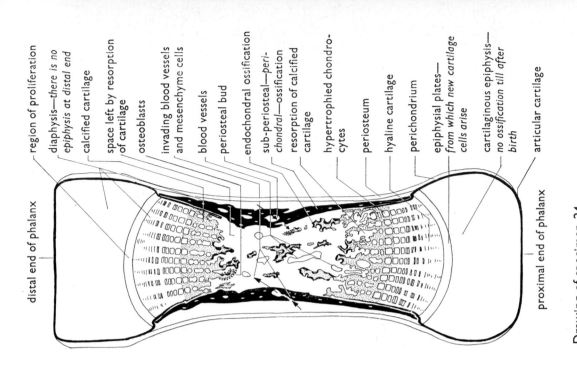

region of proliferation

diaphysis—*there is no epiphysis at distal end*

calcified cartilage

space left by resorption of cartilage

osteoblasts

invading blood vessels and mesenchyme cells

blood vessels

periosteal bud

endochondral ossification

sub-periosteal—*peri-chondral*—ossification

resorption of calcified cartilage

hypertrophied chondro-cytes

periosteum

hyaline cartilage

perichondrium

epiphysial plates—from which new cartilage cells arise

cartilaginous epiphysis—*no ossification till after birth*

articular cartilage

distal end of phalanx

proximal end of phalanx

Drawing of specimen 24

cartilage model of a phalanx

finger

distal phalanx

perichondrium

hyaline cartilage

calcified cartilage

proximal phalanx

hypertrophied chondrocytes—*these cells secrete the enzyme phosphatase which causes the matrix to calcify. This in turn brings about the death of the cells. The cells break down leaving spaces, the primary areolae*

Drawing based on specimen 23 (idealised and simplified)

31

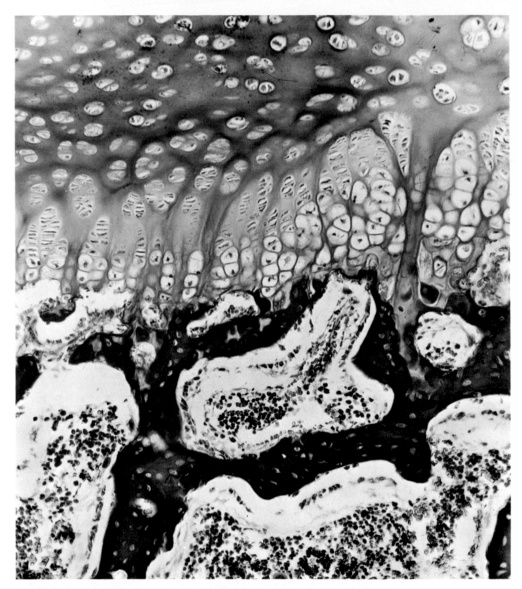

25. **Ossification,** detail, L.S. (rat vertebra, L.S.), mag. 250×

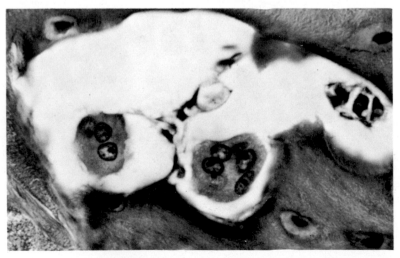

26. **Osteoclasts,** L.S. (rat spongy bone, L.S.), mag. 1000×

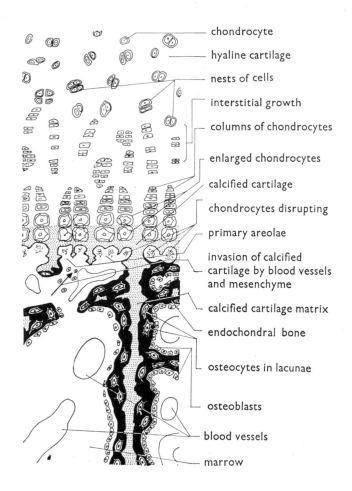

chondrocyte

hyaline cartilage

nests of cells

interstitial growth

columns of chondrocytes

enlarged chondrocytes

calcified cartilage

chondrocytes disrupting

primary areolae

invasion of calcified
cartilage by blood vessels
and mesenchyme

calcified cartilage matrix

endochondral bone

osteocytes in lacunae

osteoblasts

blood vessels

marrow

Drawing based on specimen 25 (idealised and simplified)

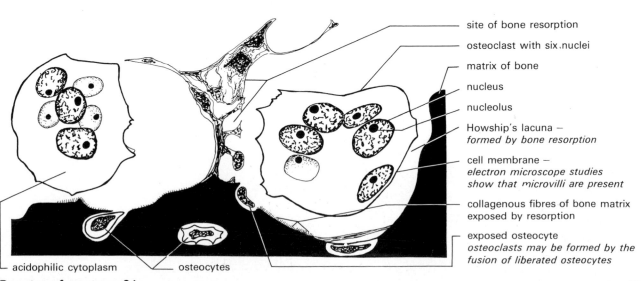

site of bone resorption

osteoclast with six nuclei

matrix of bone

nucleus

nucleolus

Howship's lacuna –
formed by bone resorption

cell membrane –
*electron microscope studies
show that microvilli are present*

collagenous fibres of bone matrix
exposed by resorption

exposed osteocyte
*osteoclasts may be formed by the
fusion of liberated osteocytes*

acidophilic cytoplasm

osteocytes

Drawing of specimen 26

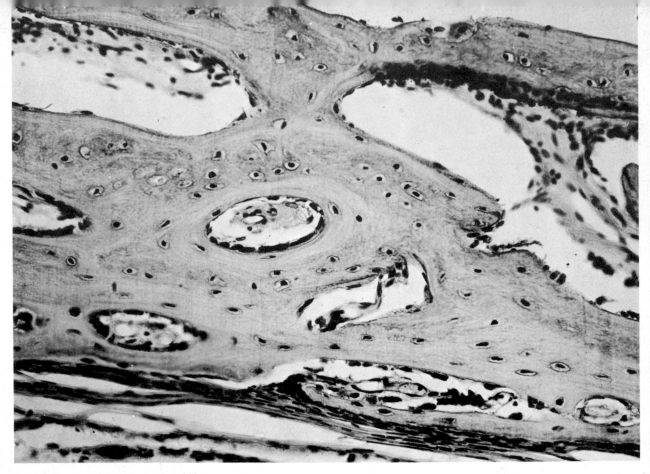

27. **Spongy bone, L.S. (rat), mag. 200×**

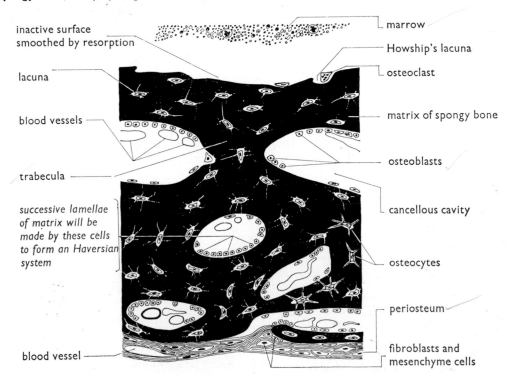

inactive surface
smoothed by resorption

marrow

Howship's lacuna

lacuna

osteoclast

blood vessels

matrix of spongy bone

osteoblasts

trabecula

cancellous cavity

*successive lamellae
of matrix will be
made by these cells
to form an Haversian
system*

osteocytes

periosteum

blood vessel

fibroblasts and
mesenchyme cells

Drawing of specimen 27

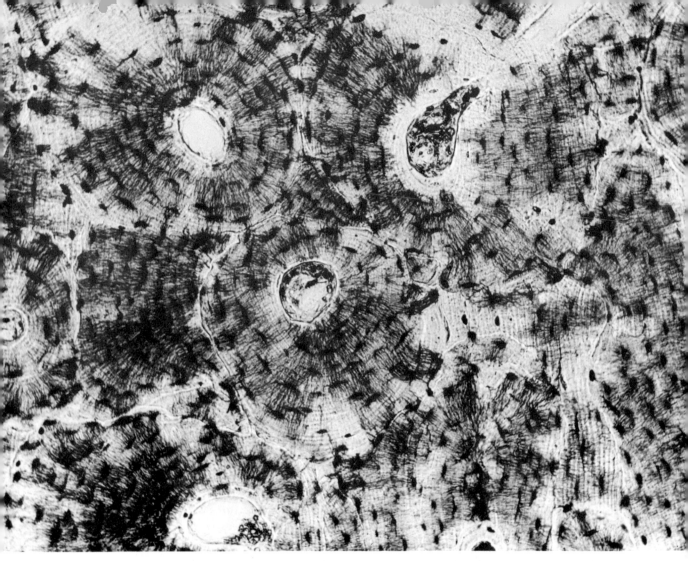

28. **Compact bone**, T.S. (human femur, T.S. ground section), mag. 100×

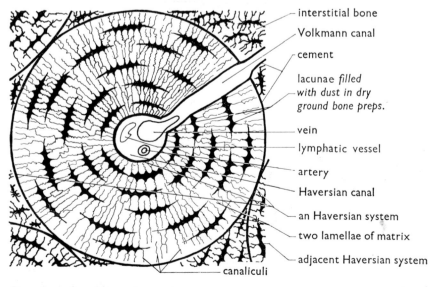

interstitial bone
Volkmann canal
cement
lacunae *filled
with dust in dry
ground bone preps.*
vein
lymphatic vessel
artery
Haversian canal
an Haversian system
two lamellae of matrix
adjacent Haversian system
canaliculi

Drawing of an Haversian system

MUSCULAR TISSUE

Muscular tissue is derived from mesoderm and is specialized for contraction. It is made up of elongated units, the muscle fibres, bound in a framework of vascular connective tissue which also provides an anchorage to the skeleton or skin.

Three different types of muscle fibre can be distinguished, each adapted to perform one special kind of contraction. Skeletal muscle contracts with rapidity during locomotion; the smooth muscle of the wall of the alimentary tract exhibits the slow rhythmic contractions of peristalsis; while the muscle of the heart continues to beat rhythmically, at a rate intermediate between that of skeletal and smooth muscle, throughout life.

The contraction of muscle fibres is brought about by a change in the arrangement of their protein molecules. The energy required is derived from the chemical energy of food.

Food and oxygen are supplied in blood circulating in an extensive network of capillaries within the muscle.

Striped muscle contracts in response to motor impulses from the central nervous system. Each motor nerve fibre has from ten to over one hundred branches each terminating at a motor end plate on a muscle fibre.

A motor axon, and the muscle fibres it serves, constitute a motor unit; the muscle fibres of one motor unit contract in unison.

Information about the length of muscle tissue is relayed to the central nervous system, from muscle spindles, which act as stretch receptors.

The sensory input from muscle spindles modifies the outgoing motor impulses.

TABLE TO COMPARE THREE TYPES OF MUSCLE FIBRES

	SMOOTH	STRIPED	CARDIAC
pseudonyms	involuntary, non-striated, unstriped, plain	voluntary, striated, striped, red and white skeletal	heart
sarcolemma (shown by electron microscopy to be a composite structure)	absent	present. Consists of plasmalemma, basement membrane, and reticular fibres	present. Structure similar to that of striped muscle
myofibrils	inconspicuous	conspicuous	fairly conspicuous
length of fibre	0.02mm to 0.5mm	1 to 40mm	0.08mm or less
diameter of fibre	8 to 10μ at thickest part	10 to 40μ	15μ approx
branching of fibre	none	none	frequent
composition of fibre	single cell	multinucleate syncytium	single branching cell
nucleus	central	many nuclei at periphery of each fibre	central
cross striations	absent	present	present
intercalated discs	absent	absent	present
contraction	slow, rhythmic, sustained	rapid, powerful; not sustained	moderately rapid, with rests between contractions. Not sustained
control of contraction	impulses from CNS not essential for contraction	neurogenic; contracts only in response to motor impulses from CNS	myogenic; but rate controlled by autonomic nervous system
distribution	alimentary, respiratory, and urogenital tracts. Blood vessels and larger lymphatics. Main ducts of glands. Ciliary muscle of eye. Arrector pili muscle of skin	locomotory muscles. Sheets of muscle of abdominal wall etc. under skin. Diaphragm, middle ear muscles	heart only

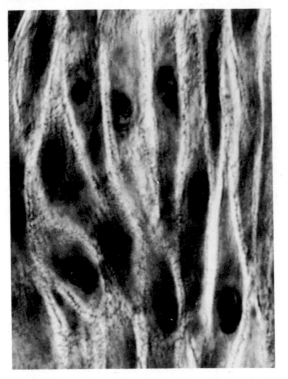

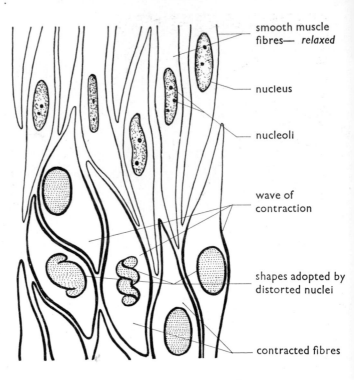

smooth muscle
fibres— *relaxed*

nucleus

nucleoli

wave of
contraction

shapes adopted by
distorted nuclei

contracted fibres

29. Smooth muscle, L.S. (rat stomach, T.S.), mag. 1100×

Drawing of specimen 29

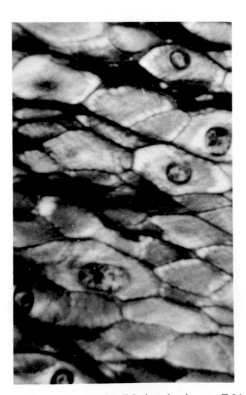

smooth muscle fibres
dovetailed together

fibre cut through widest
middle region

fibre cut near tapered end

few nuclei cut through:
nucleus central

Drawing of specimen 30

30. Smooth muscle, T.S. (cat duodenum, T.S.), mag. 1100×

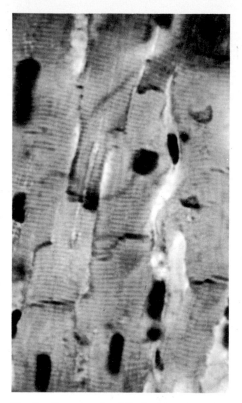

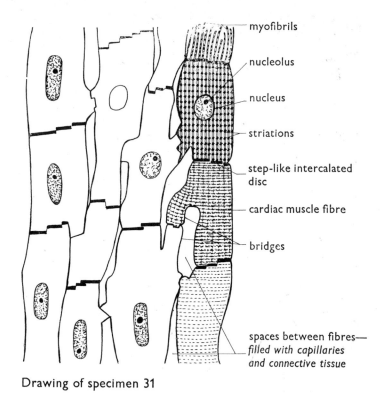

myofibrils

nucleolus

nucleus

striations

step-like intercalated disc

cardiac muscle fibre

bridges

spaces between fibres— *filled with capillaries and connective tissue*

Drawing of specimen 31

31. Cardiac muscle, L.S. (human ventricle, L.S.), mag. 1100×

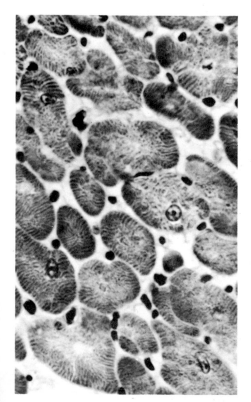

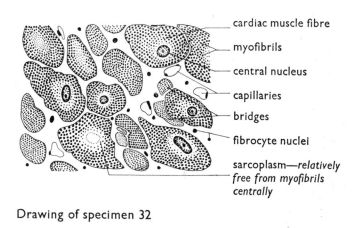

cardiac muscle fibre

myofibrils

central nucleus

capillaries

bridges

fibrocyte nuclei

sarcoplasm—*relatively free from myofibrils centrally*

Drawing of specimen 32

32. Cardiac muscle, T.S. (sheep ventricle, T.S.), mag. 1100×

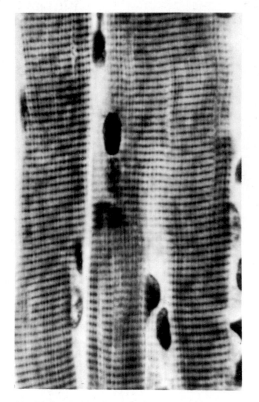
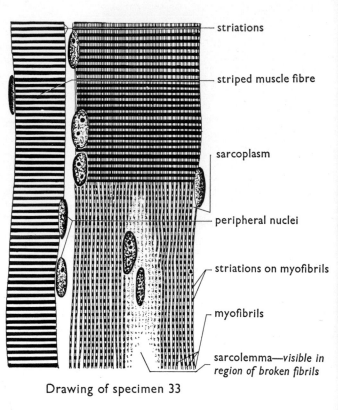

striations

striped muscle fibre

sarcoplasm

peripheral nuclei

striations on myofibrils

myofibrils

sarcolemma—*visible in region of broken fibrils*

Drawing of specimen 33

33. Striped muscle, L.S. (monkey rectus muscle, L.S.), mag. 1100×

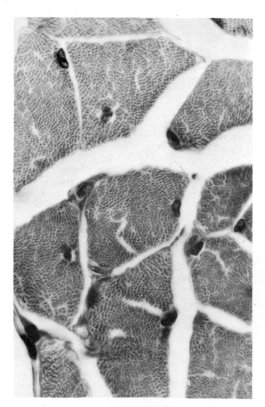
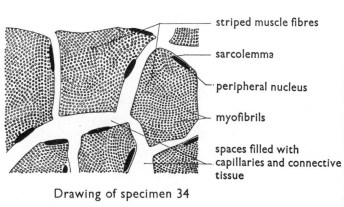

striped muscle fibres

sarcolemma

peripheral nucleus

myofibrils

spaces filled with capillaries and connective tissue

Drawing of specimen 34

34. Striped muscle, T.S. (monkey rectus muscle, T.S.), mag. 1100×

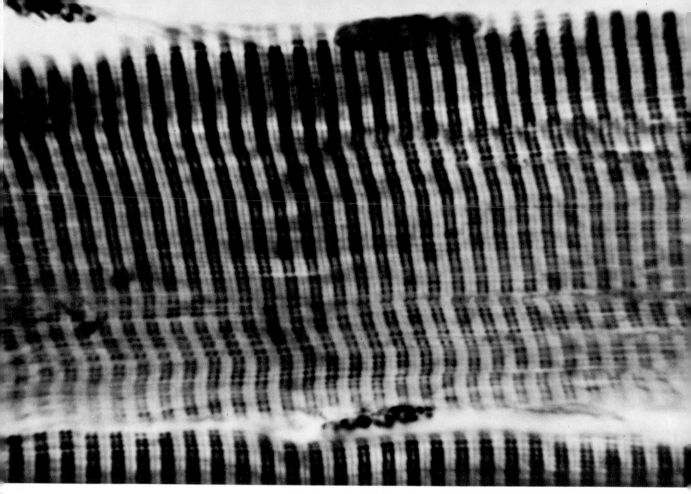

35. **Striped muscle,** L.S. for striations (monkey rectus muscle, L.S.), mag. 2400×

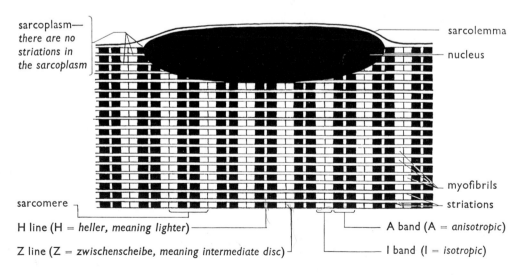

sarcoplasm—there are no striations in the sarcoplasm

sarcolemma

nucleus

myofibrils

striations

sarcomere

H line (H = *heller*, meaning lighter)

Z line (Z = *zwischenscheibe*, meaning intermediate disc)

A band (A = *anisotropic*)

I band (I = *isotropic*)

Diagram to explain specimen 35

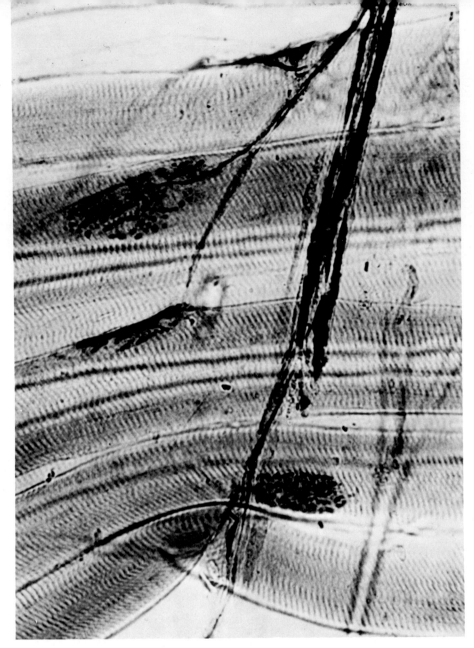

36. Motor end plates (snake muscle squash), mag. 850×

Motor end plates

The ultimate branches of a motor axon terminate in motor end plates on the surface of muscle fibres. Every striped muscle fibre has one nerve terminal. At neuro-muscular junctions muscle fibres have many nuclei but lack striations. The nerve fibre loses its medullary sheath just before entering the end plate.

It is difficult to interpret the structure of the nerve terminals even in preparations where the nerve fibres have been impregnated

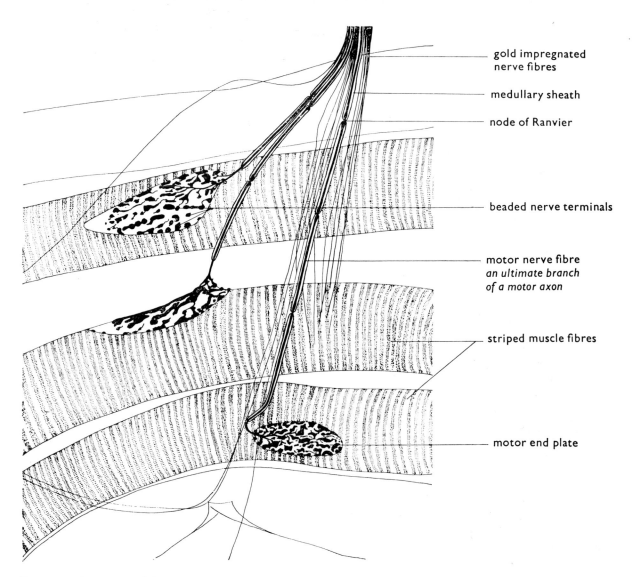

gold impregnated
nerve fibres

medullary sheath

node of Ranvier

beaded nerve terminals

motor nerve fibre
*an ultimate branch
of a motor axon*

striped muscle fibres

motor end plate

Drawing of specimen 36

with gold or silver. In many cases the nerve fibre forms a tangle of beaded branches in the end plate as can be seen in specimen 36. Electron micrographs reveal vesicles in the nerve terminals. The arrival of a nerve impulse causes the vesicles to release acetylcholine which excites the muscle fibres to contract.

Because the muscle fibres of a motor unit are dispersed throughout a muscle their contractions produce a general effect rather than a local one. The tension of a muscle depends upon the number of motor units which are active at any moment. Coarse movements such as those of a thigh muscle are performed by motor units each containing a hundred or more muscle fibres. The precise movements of extrinsic eye muscles involve motor units with as few as one or two muscle fibres.

NERVOUS TISSUE

Nervous tissue develops from embryonic ectoderm. The unit of the nervous system is the nerve cell or neurone whose specialized cytoplasm is highly irritable and conductive. Neurones provide communication units linking receptors and effectors.

A nerve cell is irritable in the sense that it can be excited by a stimulus. A stimulus can be defined as a change in the intensity of applied physico-chemical energy acting in such a way as to tend to disturb the equilibrium of living protoplasm. The energy of the stimulus is transduced into electrical energy by neurones, and this electrical energy initiates a series of events which travel along the neurone. The wave of electrical change that is conducted constitutes a nerve impulse.

Neurones conduct nerve impulses either fully or not at all, and they are capable of conduction in either direction, but normally do so only in one direction. Afferent or sensory neurones conduct impulses towards the central nervous system, while efferent or motor neurones conduct away from it.

Neurones are specialized for conduction over long distances by having processes, which may be several metres long, extending from the cell body. A distinction may be made between processes called axons which normally conduct impulses away from the cell body, and dendrons which conduct towards it.

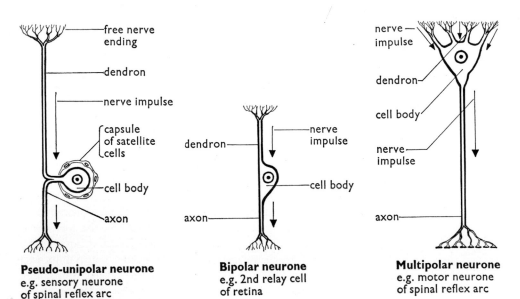

Pseudo-unipolar neurone
e.g. sensory neurone
of spinal reflex arc

Bipolar neurone
e.g. 2nd relay cell
of retina

Multipolar neurone
e.g. motor neurone
of spinal reflex arc

DIAGRAM ILLUSTRATING THE VARIOUS TYPES OF NEURONE

Nerve cells vary in the number of processes arising from them. Thus bipolar neurones have two processes while multipolar have many. A sensory neurone is described as pseudo-unipolar, since its single process is thought to consist of two closely opposed processes, although the evidence for this is not conclusive.

The processes of nerve cells are called nerve fibres. These occur in all parts of the nervous system. The white matter of brain and spinal cord is almost entirely nerve fibres; fibres are also profusely distributed throughout the grey matter. Nerves outside the central system are made up of nerve fibres supported by connective tissue.

Neurones are large cells. The nucleated part of the neurone is referred to as the cell body, the cytoplasm round the nucleus being called the perikaryon. The large spherical nucleus stains palely, but a conspicuous deeply staining nucleolus is present.

Cell bodies occur mainly in the grey matter of the central nervous system and in ganglia. Within the cytoplasm of the neurone are delicate threads, the neurofibrils, extending from the cell body into the processes. They are demonstrated by silver techniques. Varying amounts of granular chromophil material occur in the cytoplasm; this material forms Nissl's granules, which stain with toluidine blue and thionine. Nissl's granules consist of ribonucleoprotein, and are associated with protein synthesis. They extend into the dendrons but are absent from the axon hillock.

All neurones contain a reticular Golgi apparatus, but lack a centrosome. Once a nerve cell has differentiated, it loses the ability to divide; this may be related to the absence of a centrosome. Pigment granules of melanin and lipochrome are often present in neurones.

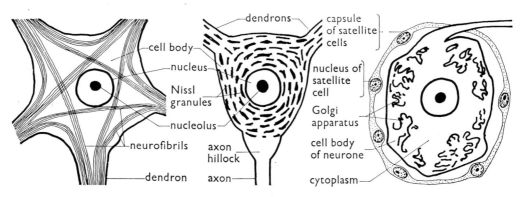

nerve cell body in a silver preparation of spinal cord of pigeon showing neurofibrils

motor neurone in a methylene blue preparation of spinal cord of cat showing Nissl granules

pseudo-unipolar neurone in a silver preparation of the dorsal root ganglion showing the Golgi apparatus

DIAGRAM TO ILLUSTRATE THE DETAILED STRUCTURE OF THE CELL BODY OF NEURONES

Nerve cells have associated with them another remarkable kind of cell, the Schwann cells. The relationship is an intimate one in which the nerve fibres are enclosed within folds of the Schwann cells. These are arranged along the length of nerve fibres, the gaps between successive cells being the nodes of Ranvier seen in medullated nerve fibres. There are no nodes in non-medullated fibres, and the nerves differ also in the number of fibres enclosed by a Schwann cell. In non-medullated nerves, as many as nine nerve fibres may be enfolded by each Schwann cell; in medullated nerves the Schwann cell wraps round a single fibre. The elaborate coiling of the Schwann cells round medullated fibres can be seen only in electron micrographs.

Schwann cells are rich in fat, hence the medullary sheath which they form appears as a dark ring round transversely cut fibres in osmic preparations.

Nerve fibres are of different diameters, and there is close correlation between thickness of fibre and speed of conduction; thick fibres conducting faster than thin. Erlanger and Gasser describe the following categories: 'A' fibres are up to 20μ in diameter. Their conduction velocities range from 90 metres/second to 2 metres/second. This group may be subdivided into categories according to the size of the action potentials. Medullated fibres of peripheral nerves belong to this group. 'B' fibres are from 1 to 5μ thick. Their conduction velocities are from 14 to 2 metres/second. The fine medullated preganglionic fibres of white rami belong to this group. 'C' fibres are from 0.4 to 1.0μ thick, and their conduction velocity is about 1 metre/second. This group includes some sensory fibres and non-medullated post-ganglionic fibres.

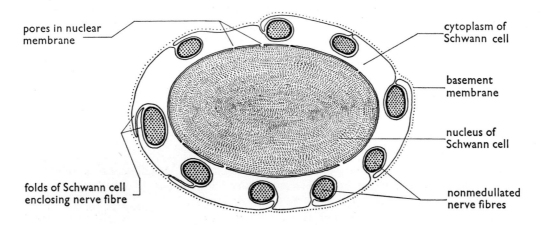

pores in nuclear membrane

cytoplasm of Schwann cell

basement membrane

nucleus of Schwann cell

folds of Schwann cell enclosing nerve fibre

nonmedullated nerve fibres

DRAWING OF NONMEDULLATED FIBRES (from an electron micrograph)

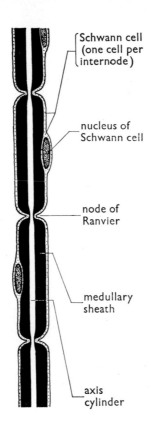

Schwann cell
(one cell per
internode)

nucleus of
Schwann cell

node of
Ranvier

DIAGRAM OF AN OSMIC
PREPARATION OF A
MEDULLATED NERVE FIBRE

medullary
sheath

axis
cylinder

Nerve endings

At its termination each nerve fibre, whether axon or dendron, has a specialized nerve ending. There are three types of these:

a. Sensory – these terminate sensory dendrons, and are specialized for the reception of stimuli. The endings may be naked, as with free nerve endings, or encapsulated as in a tactile (Meissner's) corpuscle. b. Motor. Motor axons terminate in effectors such as muscles and glands. Motor end plates are the nerve endings of motor axons in muscle fibres. c. Synapses. Every nerve cell has at least one of its sets of nerve endings associated with another nerve cell; all the nerve endings of association neurones are associated with other neurones. The region where the nerve endings of one cell come into contact with another cell is known as the synapse.

The synapse

Within the central nervous system and ganglia, each axon breaks up into fine branches with terminal swellings. These are called end-bulbs, end-feet, or boutons terminaux, and they rest on the surface of the cell body and the dendrons of the neurone with which they have a synaptic relationship. Each neurone has synaptic relationships with axons from many other neurones.

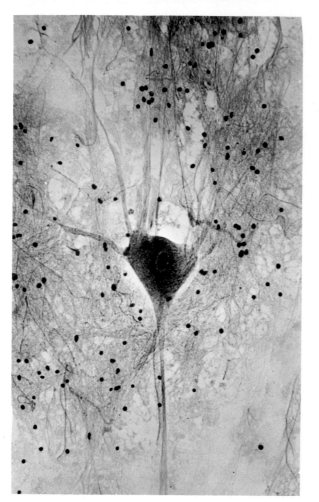

37. **Multipolar neurone** (ox spinal cord smear), mag. 200×

38. **Nodes of Ranvier,** L.S. (cat posterior root, L.S.), mag. 950×

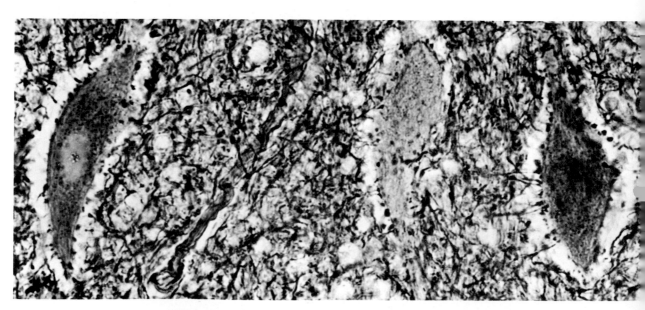

39. **Synapses** (rabbit spinal cord, T.S.), mag. 1100×

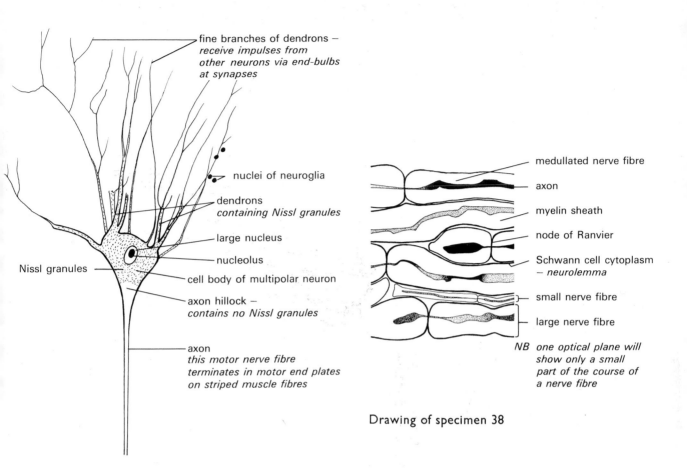

fine branches of dendrons –
*receive impulses from
other neurons via end-bulbs
at synapses*

nuclei of neuroglia

dendrons
containing Nissl granules

large nucleus

nucleolus

Nissl granules

cell body of multipolar neuron

axon hillock –
contains no Nissl granules

axon
*this motor nerve fibre
terminates in motor end plates
on striped muscle fibres*

medullated nerve fibre

axon

myelin sheath

node of Ranvier

Schwann cell cytoplasm
– *neurolemma*

small nerve fibre

large nerve fibre

*NB one optical plane will
show only a small
part of the course of
a nerve fibre*

Drawing of specimen 38

Drawing of specimen 37

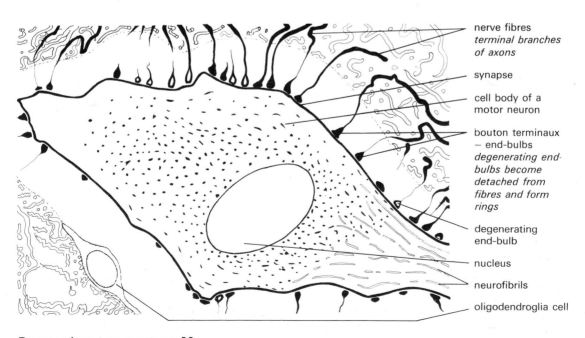

nerve fibres
*terminal branches
of axons*

synapse

cell body of a
motor neuron

bouton terminaux
– end-bulbs
*degenerating end-
bulbs become
detached from
fibres and form
rings*

degenerating
end-bulb

nucleus

neurofibrils

oligodendroglia cell

Drawing based on specimen 39

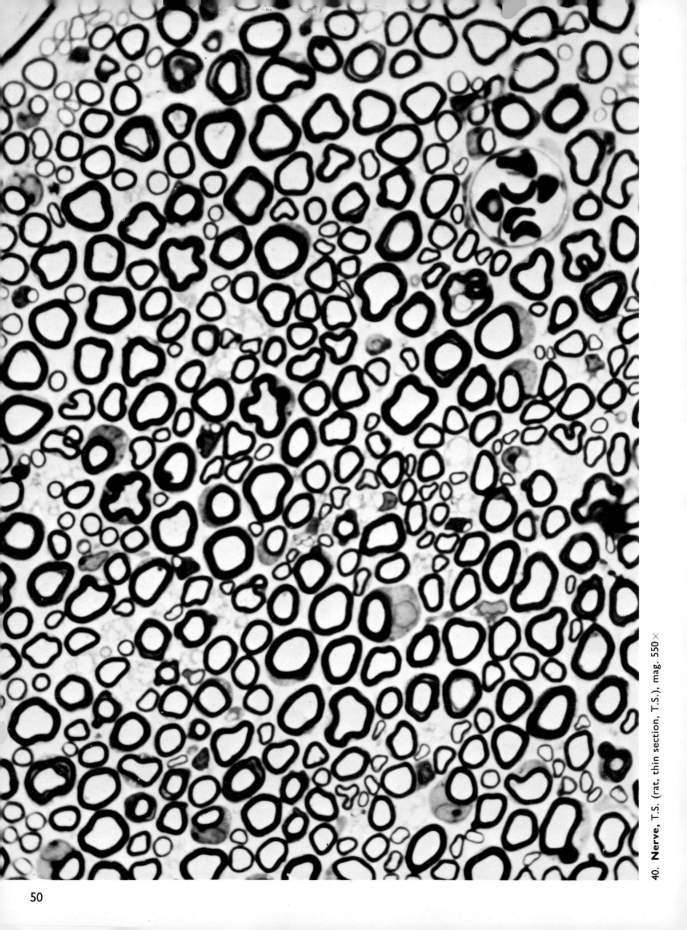

40. **Nerve**, T.S. (rat, thin section, T.S.), mag. 550×

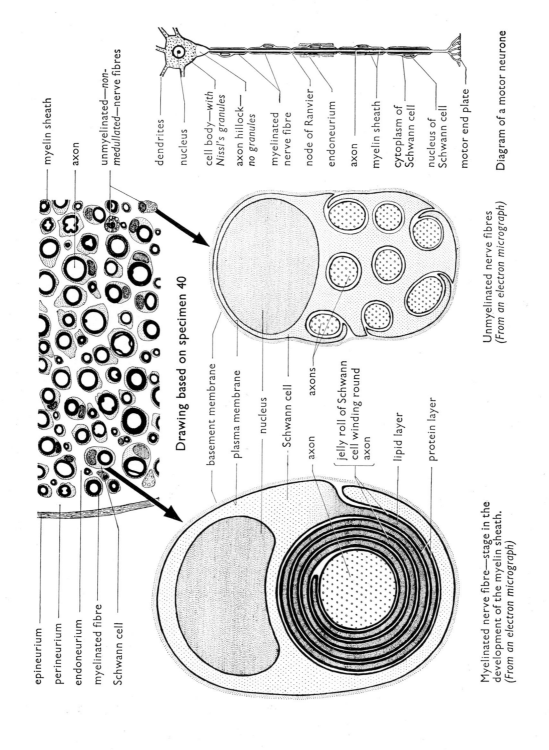

myelin sheath

axon

unmyelinated—*non-medullated*—nerve fibres

dendrites

nucleus

cell body—with *Nissl's granules*

axon hillock—*no granules*

myelinated nerve fibre

node of Ranvier

endoneurium

axon

myelin sheath

cytoplasm of Schwann cell

nucleus of Schwann cell

motor end plate

Diagram of a motor neurone

epineurium

perineurium

endoneurium

myelinated fibre

Schwann cell

Drawing based on specimen 40

basement membrane

plasma membrane

nucleus

Schwann cell

axons

Unmyelinated nerve fibres
(From an electron micrograph)

nucleus

Schwann cell

axon

jelly roll of Schwann cell winding round axon

lipid layer

protein layer

Myelinated nerve fibre—stage in the development of the myelin sheath.
(From an electron micrograph)

51

ORGAN SYSTEMS

THE DIGESTIVE SYSTEM

The digestive tract is in a sense external to the other systems, its lumen being continuous with the outside world. The lining of the tract acts in a defensive capacity. Before food can be used by the body it has to undergo mechanical and chemical changes. These changes are accomplished, stage by stage, in the various regions of the system, starting with mechanical breakdown by teeth and tongue in the buccal cavity. Food is moved from region to region by peristaltic waves of contraction of the smooth muscle fibres in the wall of the gut tube. The smooth muscle layer also provides a churning action which mixes the food with digestive juices. The chemical changes are hydrolytic and are catalysed by enzymes. The necessary water for hydrolysis is provided by copious secretion from the lining epithelium and glands of the gut. Mucus assists movement by acting as a lubricant. Digestive enzymes are secreted by glands either in the gut wall, e.g. glands of the stomach, or outside the tract, e.g. pancreas, in which case the secretion is poured into the gut along ducts.

The products of digestion, mainly soluble substances, are absorbed through the villi of the small intestine. The remaining water is absorbed principally through the wall of the large intestine.

Each region of the alimentary canal is adapted to its special functions. The special features of the regions are listed in the accompanying table. Histologically all regions exhibit a common basic plan which is illustrated in the diagram.

GENERAL HISTOLOGY OF THE ALIMENTARY CANAL

The alimentary canal may be identified by its tubular nature and the division of its wall into four distinct layers, namely:
1. *Mucosa*
2. *Submucosa*
3. *Muscularis externa*
4. *Serosa*

1. *Mucosa*. This is the innermost layer of the alimentary canal, consisting of three layers.

a. Epithelium. This layer is derived from embryonic endoderm except for the anal canal and part of the buccal cavity which are ectodermal in origin (the other layers of the wall are of mesodermal origin). All the glands of the digestive system develop from this epithelium.

b. Lamina propria. This is a layer of loose connective tissue which supports the epithelium. In most regions the lamina propria accommodates glands; it also contains blood vessels, lymphatic vessels, and may contain lymph nodes.

c. Muscularis mucosa. This constitutes the outermost layer of the mucosa; it is made up of smooth muscle fibres.

2. *Submucosa*. This is largely composed of collagenous fibres but elastic fibres are also present. The submucosa accommodates blood vessels, lymphatic vessels, nerves, and Meissner's plexus. Glands occur in the submucosa of the oesophagus and duodenum. Lymphatic tissue projects into the submucosa, particularly in the large intestine.

3. *Muscularis externa*. In most regions this is made up of an outer sheet of longitudinally arranged smooth muscle fibres and an inner sheet of circularly arranged fibres. Auerbach's plexus lies between these sheets of muscle fibres and co-ordinates their activities.

4. *Serosa*. This is a layer of areolar tissue continuous with the mesenteries supporting the gut.

DIGESTIVE SYSTEM

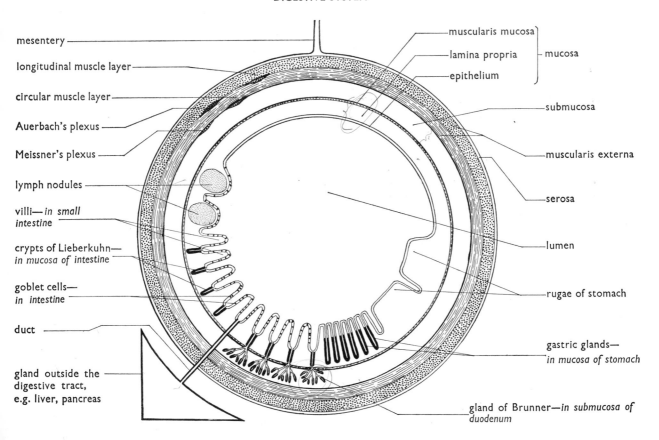

mesentery

longitudinal muscle layer

circular muscle layer

Auerbach's plexus

Meissner's plexus

lymph nodules

villi—*in small intestine*

crypts of Lieberkuhn— *in mucosa of intestine*

goblet cells— *in intestine*

duct

gland outside the digestive tract, e.g. liver, pancreas

muscularis mucosa

lamina propria — mucosa

epithelium

submucosa

muscularis externa

serosa

lumen

rugae of stomach

gastric glands— *in mucosa of stomach*

gland of Brunner—*in submucosa of duodenum*

DIAGRAM TO SHOW THE GENERAL PLAN OF THE ALIMENTARY CANAL

THE MAIN FEATURES OF THE ALIMENTARY CANAL

REGION	MUSCULARIS EXTERNA	SUBMUCOSA	MUCOSA — MUSCULARIS MUCOSA	MUCOSA — LAMINA PROPRIA	MUCOSA — SURFACE EPITHELIUM	GLANDS	DIAGNOSTIC FEATURES
OESOPHAGUS	Two layers, outer longitudinal and inner circular forming a thick muscular coat. In man, upper third has striped fibres, middle mixed, and lower third has smooth fibres.	Where muscularis mucosa absent it merges with lamina propria; elastic to allow for stretching during swallowing; contains mucous glands.	Thick; fibres longitudinally arranged. In man it is incomplete or absent from the upper third.	Rich in collagen fibres; has papillae projecting into epithelium; some glands occur here at either extremity of the oesophagus.	Stratified non-keratinised squamous type. In some mammals it is keratinised. Thrown into longitudinal folds reducing lumen to small star-shaped space.	Mucous glands in submucosa; some occur in lamina propria; few glands in man.	1. folded mucosa 2. stratified squamous epithelium 3. thick muscularis mucosa 4. absence of serosa 5. thickest muscularis externa 6. papillae project into epithelium
STOMACH	Three layers, outer longitudinal, middle circular, inner oblique. Oblique layer not continuous and is absent in pyloric region.	Forms large part of substance of folds (rugae).	Two layers; outer longitudinal and inner circular. Some fibres pass up between glands to be attached to epithelial basement membrane.	Loose connective tissue reduced in amount by closely-packed glands; contains some lymph nodules.	Simple columnar type; all cells alike, i.e. mucus-secreting. Gastric pits dip down to glands.	Fairly long and close together, confined to lamina propria. 3 types: 1. Cardiac, compound tubular, mucus secreting. 2. Fundic, simple branched tubular: chief, parietal, and mucous neck cells; secrete pepsinogen, rennin, mucus and HCl. 3. Pyloric; simple branched tubular; secrete mucus and possibly some enzymes.	1. rugae 2. thick wall 3. gastric pits 4. uniform epithelium 5. abundant glands in lamina propria 6. parietal cells in fundus 7. oblique layer in muscularis externa 8. no goblet cells 9. no villi
DUODENUM (the duodenum, jejunum, and ileum together constitute the small intestine).	Two layers, an outer longitudinal and an inner circular.	Raised up into folds — the plicae circulares which do not disappear on stretching; plicae low; glands of Brunner.	Two layers; thin.	Projects into villi; contains characteristic capillary bed in villi; central lacteal in villi; smooth muscle fibres; glands (crypts) present. Some lymph nodules.	Simple columnar type; 2 kinds of cells: 1. Columnar, with terminal bars and striated border. 2. Goblet, secrete mucus. Glands called crypts of Lieberkühn opening between villi; shorter than glands of stomach mucosa.	Glands of Brunner in submucosa; crypts in mucosa. Crypts have Paneth cells and argentaffin cells; they secrete digestive enzymes.	1. villi 2. two kinds of cells in epithelium 3. goblet cells 4. plicae 5. crypts 6. abundant villi (cf. jejunum and ileum) 7. short leafshaped villi 8. glands of Brunner
JEJUNUM	As for duodenum	Raised up into the tallest plicae of small intestine; very vascular.	As for duodenum.	As for duodenum.	As for duodenum.	Crypts only, no glands of Brunner.	1 to 5 – as for duodenum 6. villi less abundant 7. tongue-shaped villi with swollen ends 8. tall plicae

ILEUM (the histological differences between jejunum and ileum are slight).	As for duodenum	Fewer plicae, none in lower region. Peyer's patches extend into submucosa in places.	As for duodenum.	As for duodenum, except for lymph nodules which are aggregated together as Peyer's patches.	As for duodenum.	As for jejunum.	1 to 5 – as for duodenum 6. villi less abundant still 7. finger-shaped villi 8. plicae few or none 9. Peyer's patches
COLON	Two layers, an outer longitudinal and an inner circular. Three bands of fibres occur in longitudinal layer, the taeniae. These are equally spaced apart (120° in cross section) but are shorter than colon. Except for taeniae the muscularis layer is thin.	No plicae; lymph nodules may project into submucosa.	As for duodenum.	Thicker than in small intestine; no villi; numerous tubular glands; large lymph nodules.	Simple columnar; very few goblet cells present.	Simple tubular glands (crypts of Lieberkühn) in lamina propria, regularly arranged in rows; profusion of goblet cells characteristic feature; glands longer than those of stomach or small intestine; glands secrete mucus.	1. no villi 2. few goblet cells in epithelium 3. long tubular glands 4. abundant goblet cells in glands 5. taeniae (in LS they may be cut along their length or not at all) 6. thin muscularis externa 7. large lumen 8. Peyer's patches project into submucosa
APPENDIX	As for duodenum	Lymphatic tissue projects into the submucosa.	Not well developed; may be absent in places.	Contains large amount of lymphatic tissue which may form a continuous circular zone. Eosinophilic leucocytes plentiful.	Simple columnar; few goblet cells present.	Crypts fewer; goblet cells sparsely scattered.	1. ring of lymphatic tissue 2. narrow lumen (may be obliterated) 3. lymphocytes between crypts
RECTUM	No taeniae: layer much thicker than in colon.	A few isolated lymph nodules; small veins in anal canal may dilate and bulge into lumen as haemorrhoids.	Absent in anal canal; lamina propria and submucosa merge here; well-developed in rectum.	Thicker than in colon.	Becomes stratified squamous towards recto-anal junction; thrown into longitudinal folds.	As for colon except for size of glands, which are largest of alimentary canal. Glands absent in junction zone.	1 to 4 – as for colon 5. no taeniae 6. thick muscularis externa 7. longest glands 8. epithelium becomes stratified near recto-anal junction

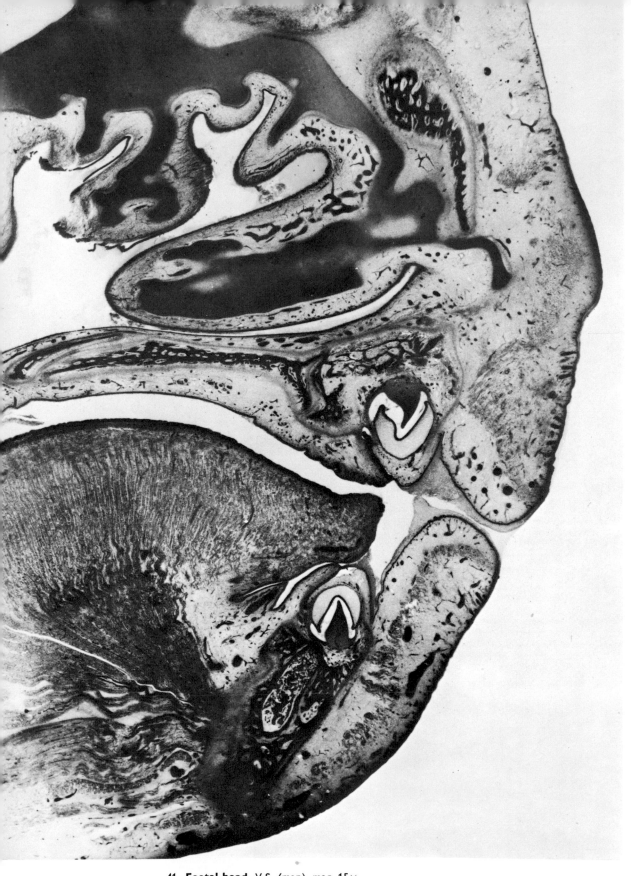

41. Foetal head, V.S. (man), mag. 15×

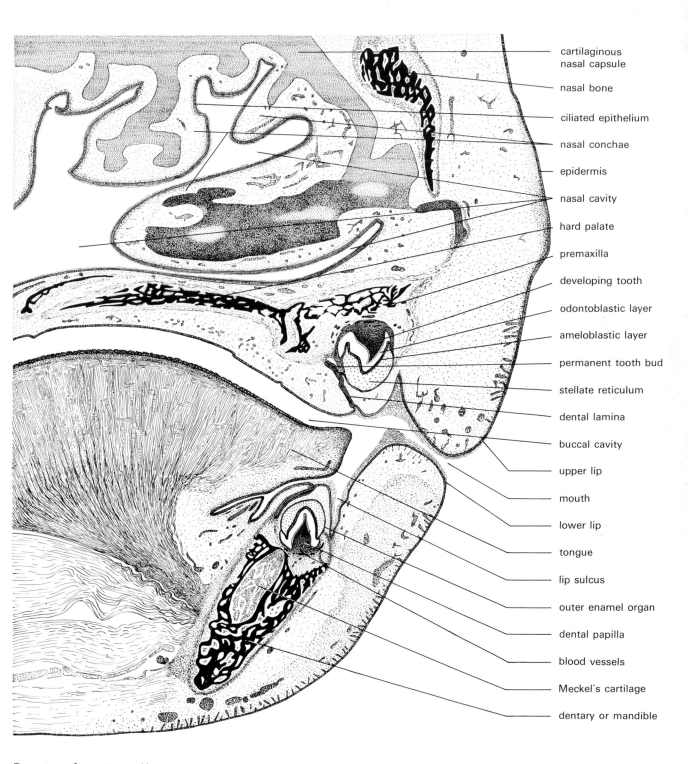

cartilaginous nasal capsule

nasal bone

ciliated epithelium

nasal conchae

epidermis

nasal cavity

hard palate

premaxilla

developing tooth

odontoblastic layer

ameloblastic layer

permanent tooth bud

stellate reticulum

dental lamina

buccal cavity

upper lip

mouth

lower lip

tongue

lip sulcus

outer enamel organ

dental papilla

blood vessels

Meckel's cartilage

dentary or mandible

Drawing of specimen 41

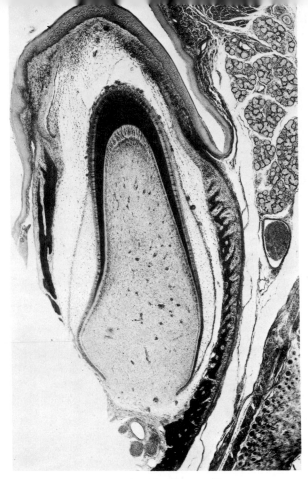

42. Developing tooth, L.S. (man), mag. 20×

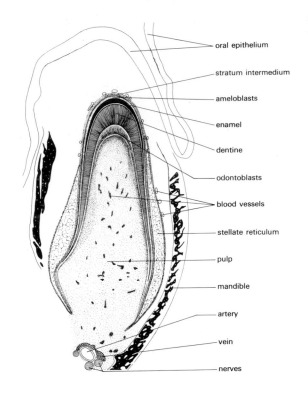

oral epithelium

stratum intermedium

ameloblasts

enamel

dentine

odontoblasts

blood vessels

stellate reticulum

pulp

mandible

artery

vein

nerves

Drawing of specimen 42

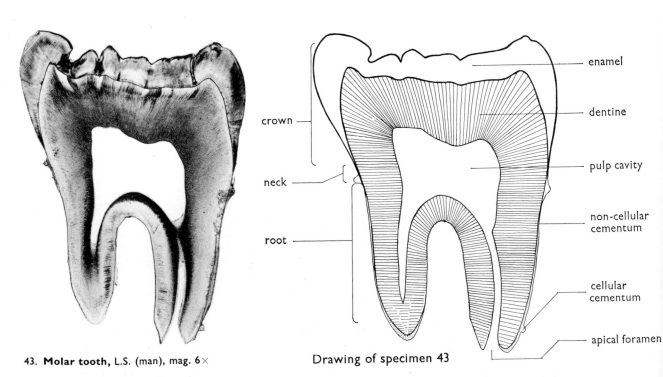

43. Molar tooth, L.S. (man), mag. 6×

crown

neck

root

enamel

dentine

pulp cavity

non-cellular cementum

cellular cementum

apical foramen

Drawing of specimen 43

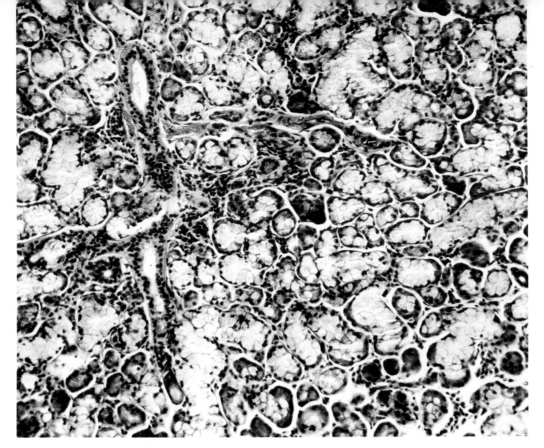

44. Sublingual gland, T.S. (man), mag. 150×

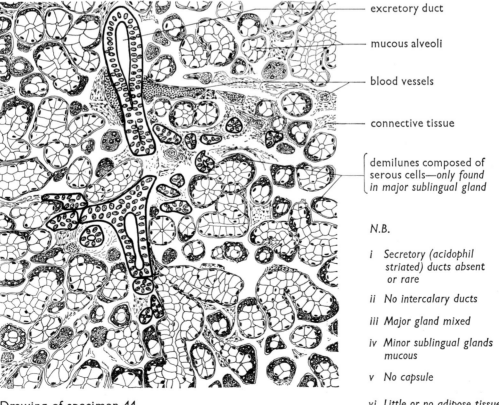

excretory duct

mucous alveoli

blood vessels

connective tissue

demilunes composed of
serous cells—*only found
in major sublingual gland*

N.B.

*i Secretory (acidophil
striated) ducts absent
or rare*

ii No intercalary ducts

iii Major gland mixed

*iv Minor sublingual glands
mucous*

v No capsule

vi Little or no adipose tissue

Drawing of specimen 44

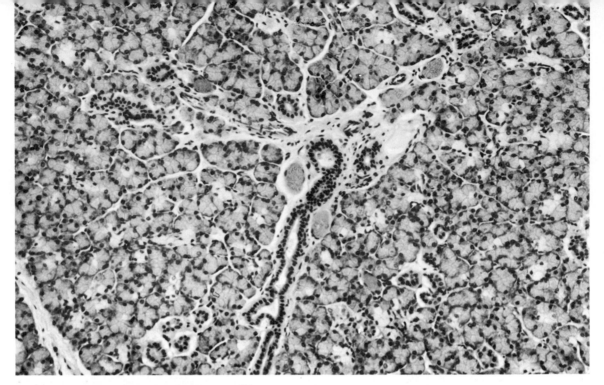

45. Submandibular gland, T.S. (man), mag. 150×

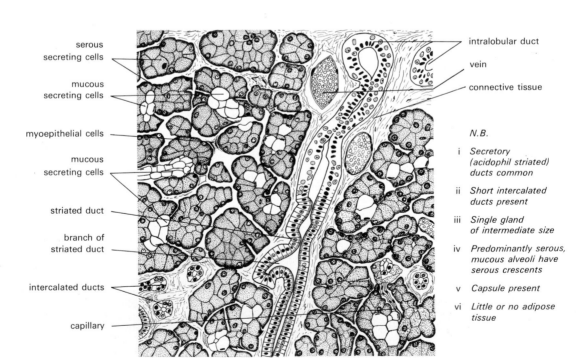

serous
secreting cells

mucous
secreting cells

myoepithelial cells

mucous
secreting cells

striated duct

branch of
striated duct

intercalated ducts

capillary

intralobular duct

vein

connective tissue

N.B.

i   *Secretory*
    (acidophil striated)
    ducts common

ii *Short intercalated*
    ducts present

iii *Single gland*
    of intermediate size

iv *Predominantly serous,*
    mucous alveoli have
    serous crescents

v   *Capsule present*

vi *Little or no adipose*
    tissue

Drawing of specimen 45

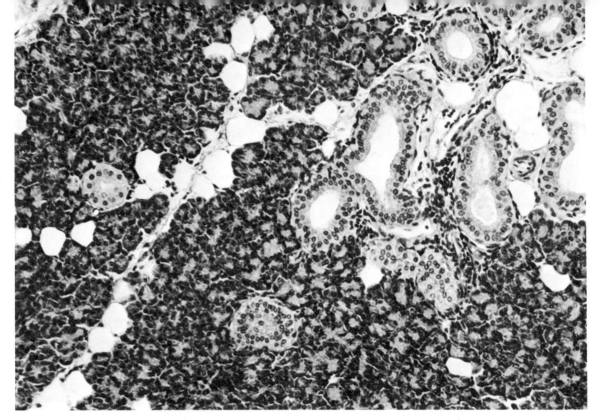

46. Parotid gland, T.S. (man), mag. 150×

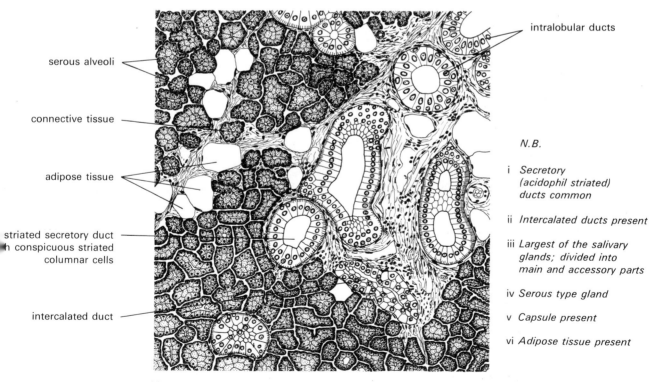

intralobular ducts

serous alveoli

connective tissue

adipose tissue

striated secretory duct
h conspicuous striated
columnar cells

intercalated duct

N.B.

i *Secretory
   (acidophil striated)
   ducts common*

ii *Intercalated ducts present*

iii *Largest of the salivary
    glands; divided into
    main and accessory parts*

iv *Serous type gland*

v *Capsule present*

vi *Adipose tissue present*

Drawing of specimen 46

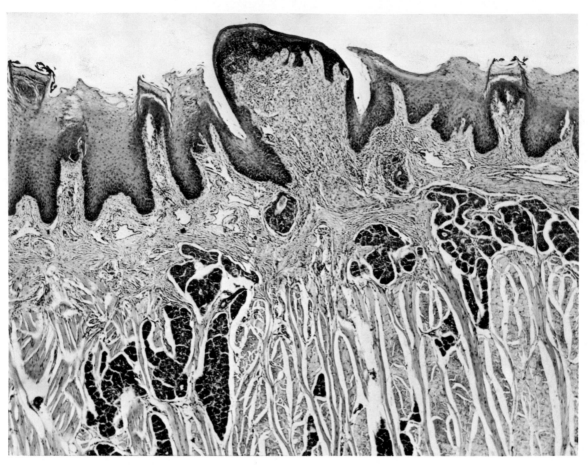

47. **Tongue,** V.S. (man), mag. 40×

48. **Taste buds,** V.S. (man, tongue, L.S.), mag. 900×

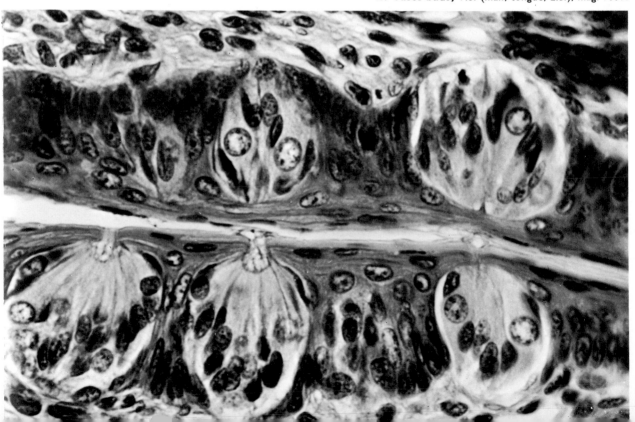

Distribution of Taste Buds

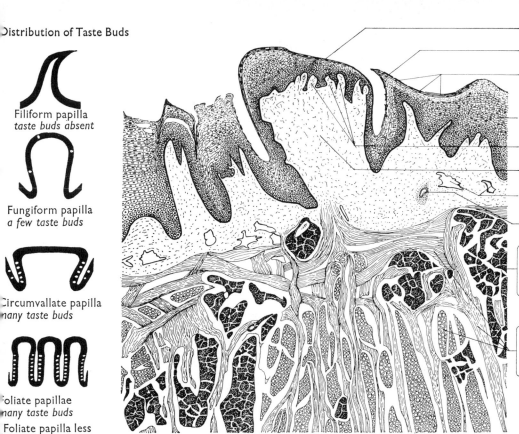

Filiform papilla
taste buds absent

Fungiform papilla
a few taste buds

Circumvallate papilla
many taste buds

Foliate papillae
many taste buds

Foliate papilla less
pronounced in man,
conspicuous in rabbit)

- fungiform papilla
- filiform papilla
- hard—*but non-keratinised
  scales which are shed*
- stratified squamous
  epithelium
- secondary papillae
- primary papilla
- blood vessels
- duct of lingual gland
- lingual gland—*serous type
  = gland of von Ebner, ducts
  open into moats of circumvallate papillae*
- striated muscle fibres—
  *the fibres are arranged
  in vertical, transverse
  and longitudinal bundles*

N.B. *There is no distinct
submucosa in the tongue*

Drawing of specimen 47

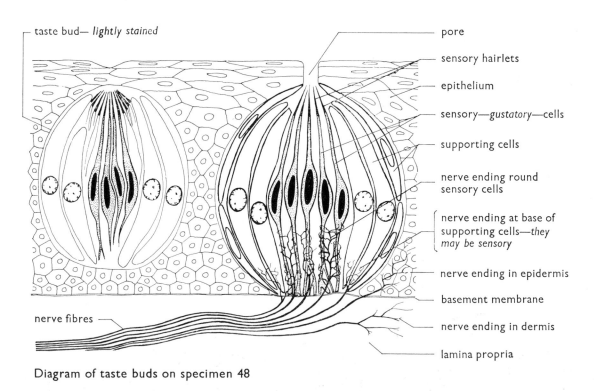

- taste bud— *lightly stained*
- nerve fibres
- pore
- sensory hairlets
- epithelium
- sensory—*gustatory*—cells
- supporting cells
- nerve ending round
  sensory cells
- nerve ending at base of
  supporting cells—*they
  may be sensory*
- nerve ending in epidermis
- basement membrane
- nerve ending in dermis
- lamina propria

Diagram of taste buds on specimen 48

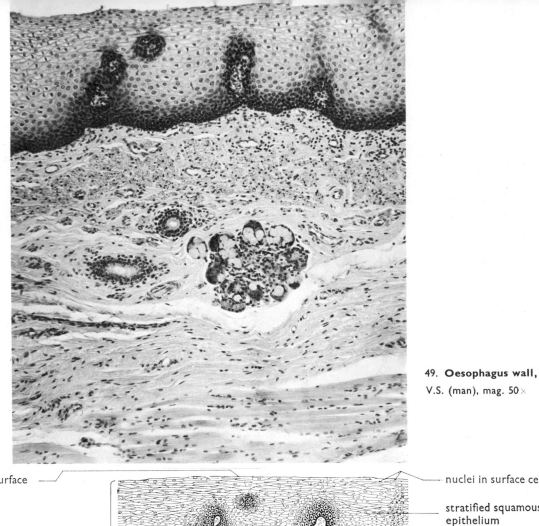

49. Oesophagus wall,
V.S. (man), mag. 50×

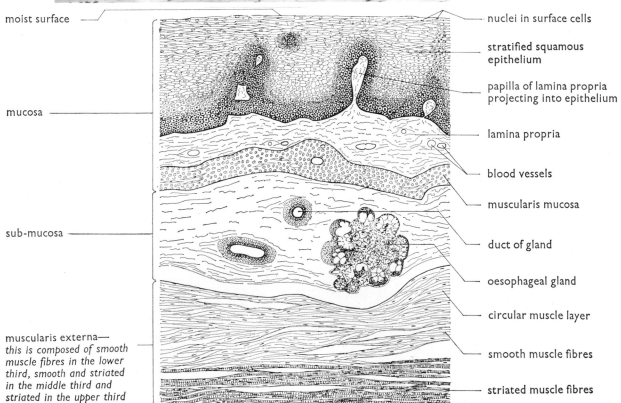

moist surface — nuclei in surface cells

stratified squamous epithelium

papilla of lamina propria projecting into epithelium

mucosa — lamina propria

blood vessels

muscularis mucosa

sub-mucosa — duct of gland

oesophageal gland

circular muscle layer

muscularis externa—
this is composed of smooth muscle fibres in the lower third, smooth and striated in the middle third and striated in the upper third

smooth muscle fibres

striated muscle fibres

Drawing of specimen 49

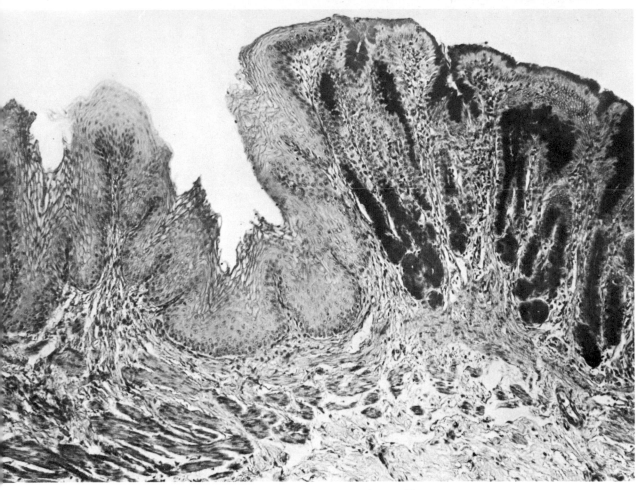

50. **Oesophagus/cardiac stomach junction,** L.S. (mammal), mag. 90 ×

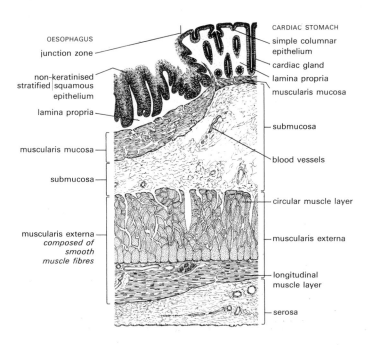

OESOPHAGUS

CARDIAC STOMACH

junction zone

simple columnar
epithelium

non-keratinised
stratified squamous
epithelium

cardiac gland

lamina propria

muscularis mucosa

lamina propria

submucosa

muscularis mucosa

blood vessels

submucosa

circular muscle layer

muscularis externa
*composed of
smooth
muscle fibres*

muscularis externa

longitudinal
muscle layer

serosa

Drawing based on specimen 50

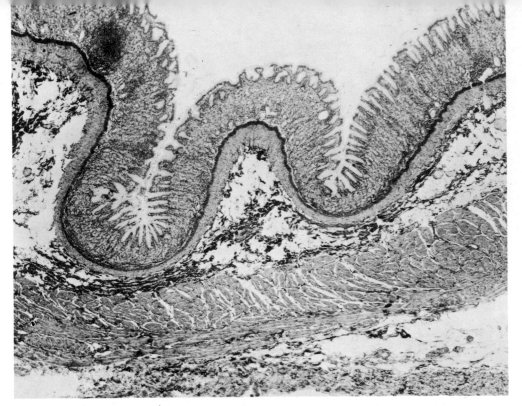

51. **Cardiac stomach wall,** L.S. (man), mag. 45×

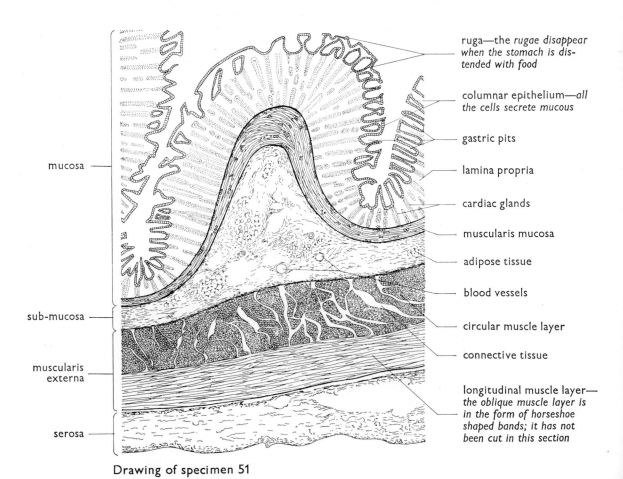

ruga—the *rugae disappear when the stomach is distended with food*

columnar epithelium—*all the cells secrete mucous*

gastric pits

lamina propria

cardiac glands

muscularis mucosa

adipose tissue

blood vessels

circular muscle layer

connective tissue

longitudinal muscle layer—*the oblique muscle layer is in the form of horseshoe shaped bands; it has not been cut in this section*

mucosa

sub-mucosa

muscularis externa

serosa

68

Drawing of specimen 51

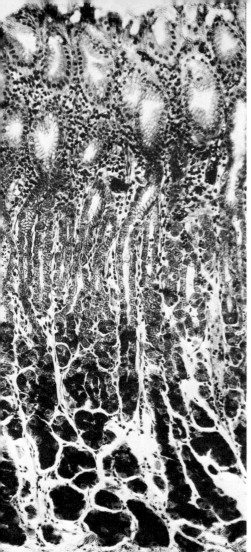

52. **Fundic stomach,** L.S. mucosa (man), mag. 100×

Diagram of a fundic gland

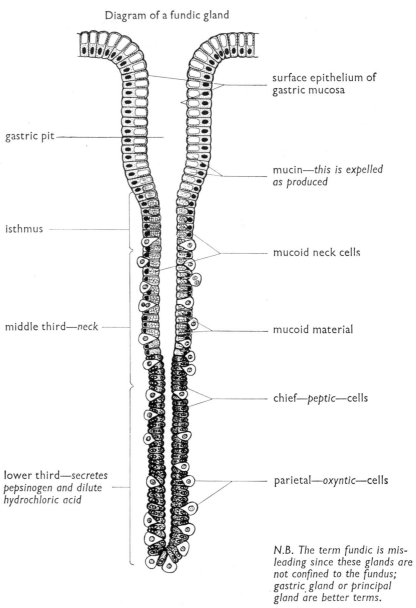

surface epithelium of gastric mucosa

gastric pit

mucin—*this is expelled as produced*

isthmus

mucoid neck cells

middle third—*neck*

mucoid material

chief—*peptic*—cells

lower third—*secretes pepsinogen and dilute hydrochloric acid*

parietal—*oxyntic*—cells

N.B. *The term fundic is misleading since these glands are not confined to the fundus; gastric gland or principal gland are better terms.*

Diagram of a reconstruction of a fundic gland based on specimen 52

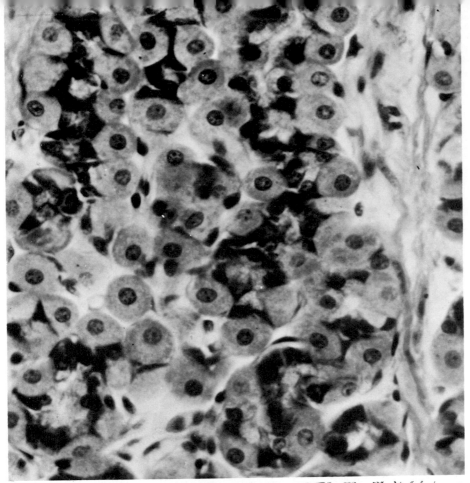

53. **Fundic gland,**
L.S. (man), mag. 850×

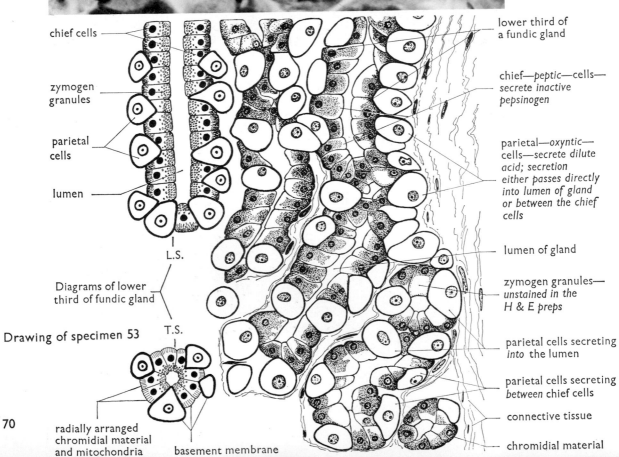

chief cells

zymogen
granules

parietal
cells

lumen

L.S.

Diagrams of lower
third of fundic gland

Drawing of specimen 53

T.S.

radially arranged
chromidial material
and mitochondria

basement membrane

lower third of
a fundic gland

chief—*peptic*—cells—
*secrete inactive
pepsinogen*

parietal—*oxyntic*—
cells—*secrete dilute
acid; secretion
either passes directly
into lumen of gland
or between the chief
cells*

lumen of gland

zymogen granules—
*unstained in the
H & E preps*

parietal cells secreting
into the lumen

parietal cells secreting
between chief cells

connective tissue

chromidial material

70

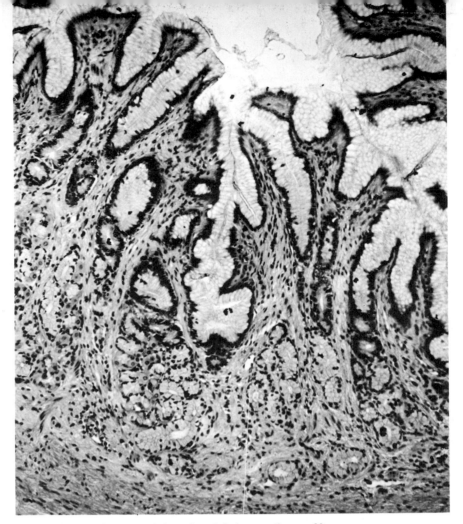

54. Fundic/pyloric stomach junction, L.S. (mammal), mag. 80×

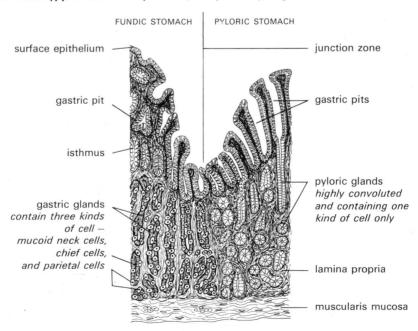

FUNDIC STOMACH | PYLORIC STOMACH

surface epithelium — junction zone

gastric pit — gastric pits

isthmus

pyloric glands
*highly convoluted
and containing one
kind of cell only*

gastric glands
*contain three kinds
of cell —
mucoid neck cells,
chief cells,
and parietal cells*

lamina propria

muscularis mucosa

Drawing based on specimen 54

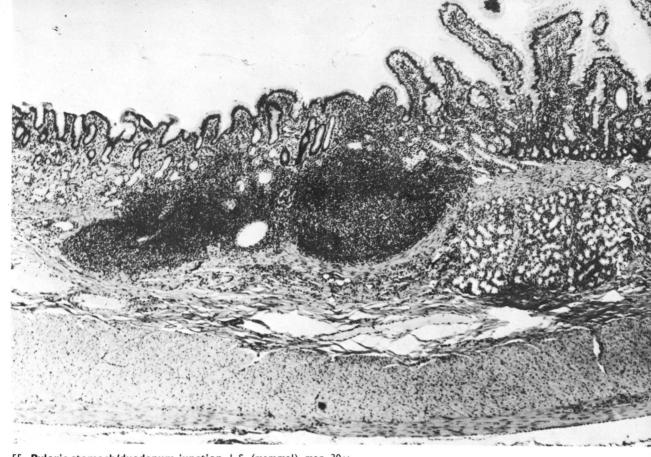

55. **Pyloric stomach/duodenum junction**, L.S. (mammal), mag. 30×

PYLORIC STOMACH   DUODENUM

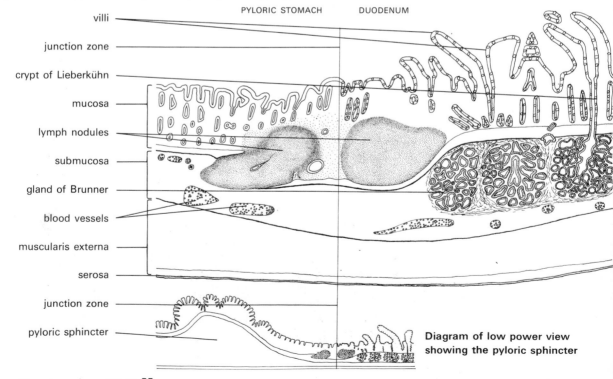

villi

junction zone

crypt of Lieberkühn

mucosa

lymph nodules

submucosa

gland of Brunner

blood vessels

muscularis externa

serosa

junction zone

pyloric sphincter

Diagram of low power view
showing the pyloric sphincter

Drawing of specimen 55

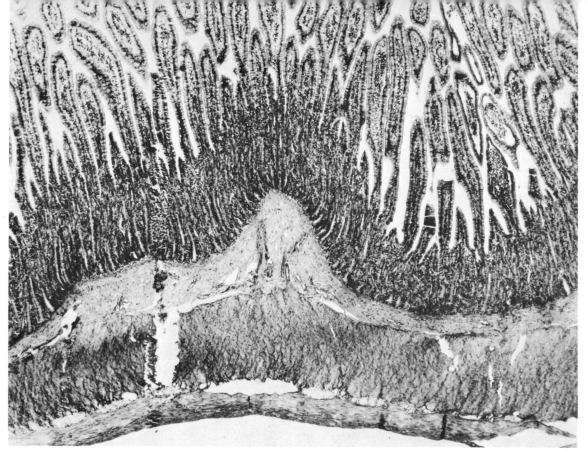

56. **Ileum,** L.S. (man), mag. 30×

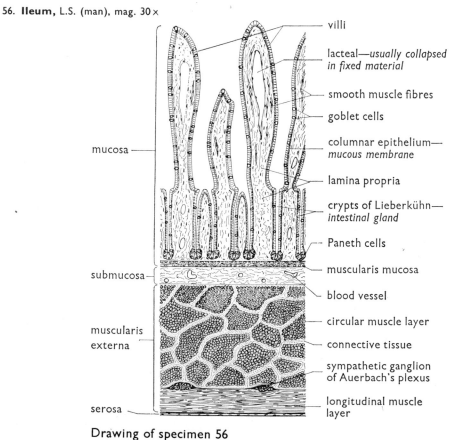

mucosa

villi

lacteal—*usually collapsed in fixed material*

smooth muscle fibres

goblet cells

columnar epithelium— *mucous membrane*

lamina propria

crypts of Lieberkühn— *intestinal gland*

Paneth cells

submucosa

muscularis mucosa

blood vessel

muscularis externa

circular muscle layer

connective tissue

sympathetic ganglion of Auerbach's plexus

serosa

longitudinal muscle layer

Drawing of specimen 56

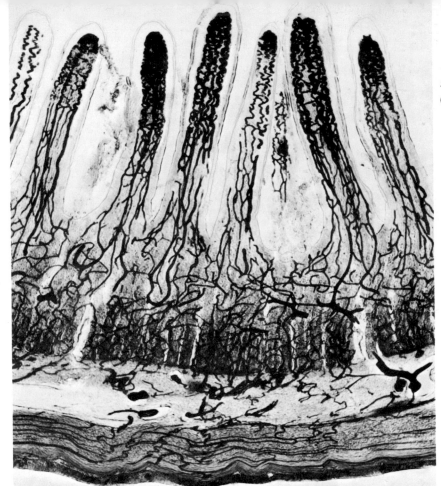

57. **Ileum,** injected blood vessels,
(cat), mag. 70×

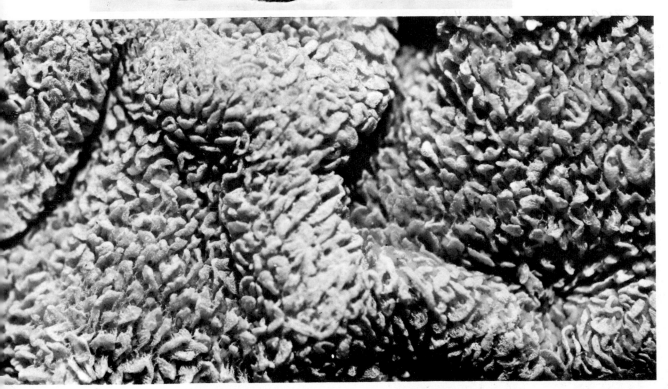

58. **Villi,** injected, surface view (human duodenum), mag. 18×

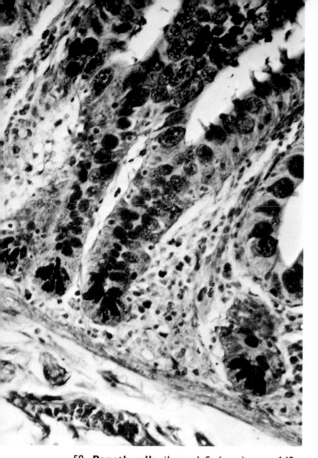

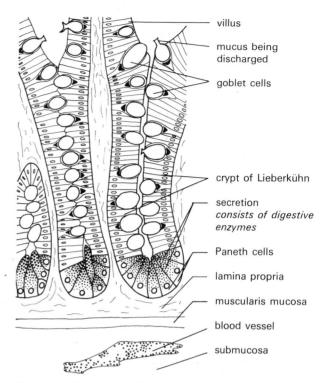

villus

mucus being
discharged

goblet cells

crypt of Lieberkühn

secretion
*consists of digestive
enzymes*

Paneth cells

lamina propria

muscularis mucosa

blood vessel

submucosa

59. **Paneth cells,** ileum, L.S. (man), mag. 140×

Drawing of specimen 59

60. **Colon,** L.S. (man), mag. 40×

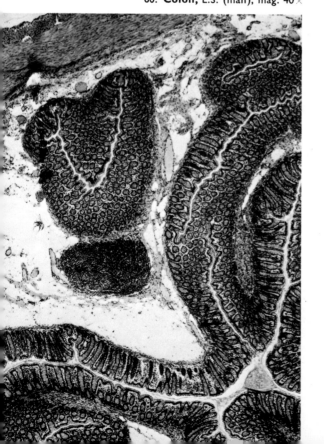

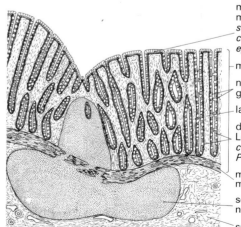

mucous
membrane
*smooth simple
columnar
epithelium*

mucosa

numerous
goblet cells

lamina propria

deep crypts of
Lieberkühn
*contain no
Paneth cells*

muscularis
mucosa

solitary lymph
nodule

submucosa

Drawing based on specimen 60

75

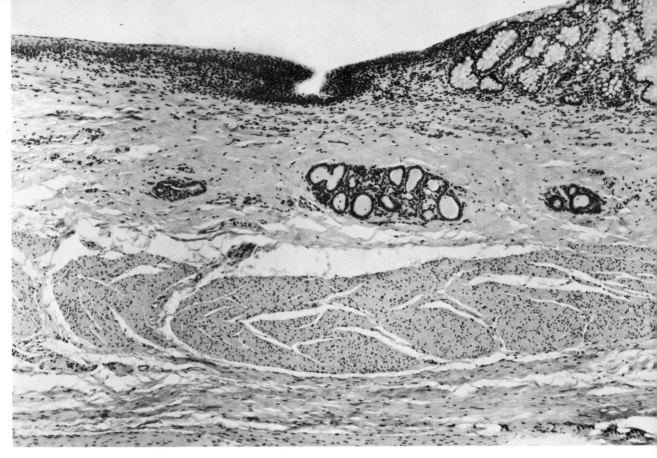

61. Recto-anal junction, L.S. (mammal), mag. 50×

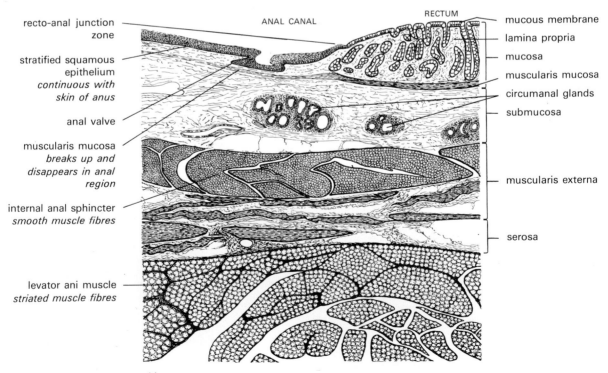

recto-anal junction zone

stratified squamous epithelium *continuous with skin of anus*

anal valve

muscularis mucosa *breaks up and disappears in anal region*

internal anal sphincter *smooth muscle fibres*

levator ani muscle *striated muscle fibres*

ANAL CANAL

RECTUM

mucous membrane

lamina propria

mucosa

muscularis mucosa

circumanal glands

submucosa

muscularis externa

serosa

Drawing of specimen 61

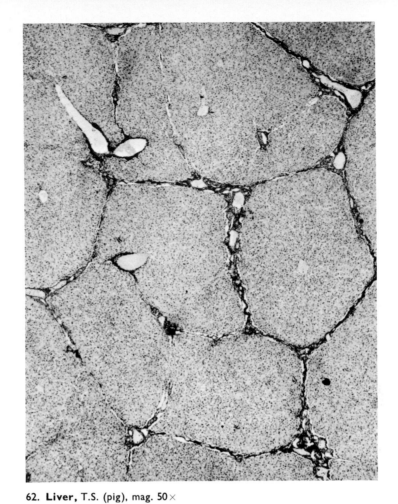

62. Liver, T.S. (pig), mag. 50×

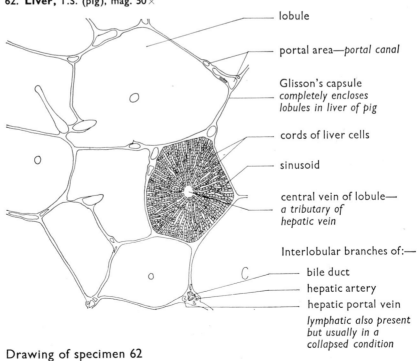

lobule

portal area—*portal canal*

Glisson's capsule
*completely encloses
lobules in liver of pig*

cords of liver cells

sinusoid

central vein of lobule—
*a tributary of
hepatic vein*

Interlobular branches of:—

bile duct
hepatic artery
hepatic portal vein
*lymphatic also present
but usually in a
collapsed condition*

Drawing of specimen 62

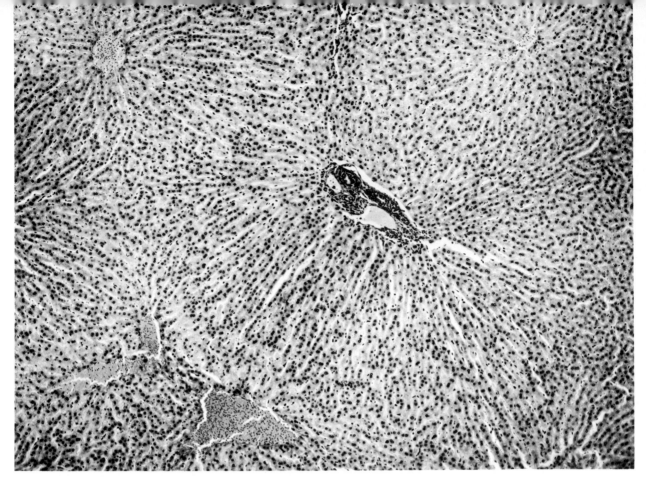

63. **Liver,** portal area, T.S. (man), mag. 120 ×

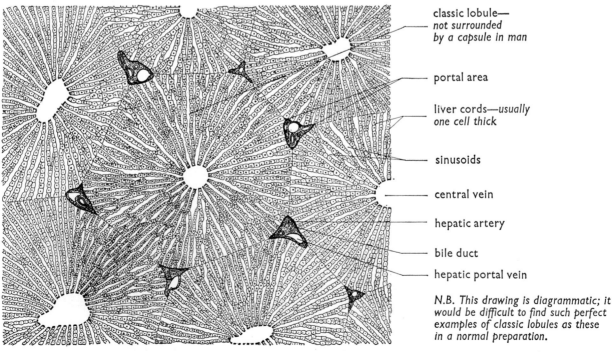

classic lobule— *not surrounded by a capsule in man*

portal area

liver cords—*usually one cell thick*

sinusoids

central vein

hepatic artery

bile duct

hepatic portal vein

N.B. This drawing is diagrammatic; it would be difficult to find such perfect examples of classic lobules as these in a normal preparation.

An interpretation of a section of human liver based upon the classic lobule concept

The classic hepatic lobule

The classic lobule is a subdivision of a liver lobe demarcated by a boundary of connective tissue. In pig's liver, the lobules have 5 or 6 sides and are about 1 mm wide and 2 mm long. A branch of the hepatic vein lies at the centre of each lobule. At the corners the connective tissue capsule encloses branches of the hepatic portal vein, the hepatic artery, bile duct and lymphatic duct; this region is known as a portal area.

The portal lobule

In the liver of man there are no sheets of connective tissue to mark off lobules. To apply the classic lobule concept necessitates finding 6 portal areas arranged about a central vein. An imaginary line through these areas would mark the boundary of a lobule. The drawing of specimen 63 illustrates this kind of interpretation. Such an arrangement is rarely if ever observed.

The usual pattern is 2 or 3 portal areas around each central vein. The region from which secretion is collected by the bile duct of one portal area is known as a portal lobule. The portal lobule is a functional unit which can be used in connection with liver physiology and pathology.

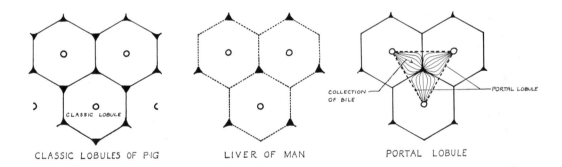

CLASSIC LOBULES OF PIG   LIVER OF MAN   PORTAL LOBULE

The interpretation of sections of the liver of man

Transverse sections of lobules are rarely encountered; this is because the lobules lie at various angles relative to each other. A further difficulty is presented by the oblique courses of the blood vessels arising from the portal areas.

It is impossible to reconstruct the structure of the liver from a transverse section. According to Elias liver cells are arranged in sheets not cords as was formerly believed. A three-dimensional figure based on the muralium theory of Elias should be consulted before attempting to interpret liver sections.

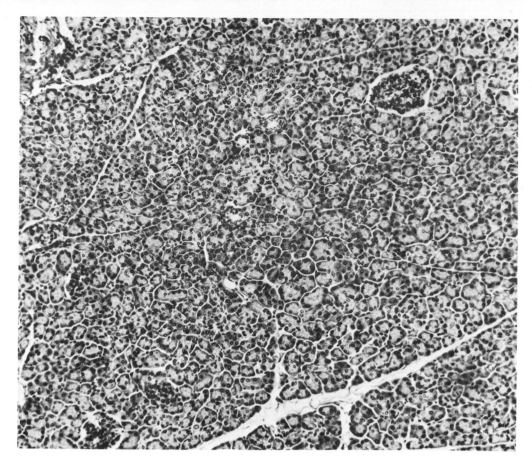

64. **Pancreas,** T.S. (monkey), mag. 65×

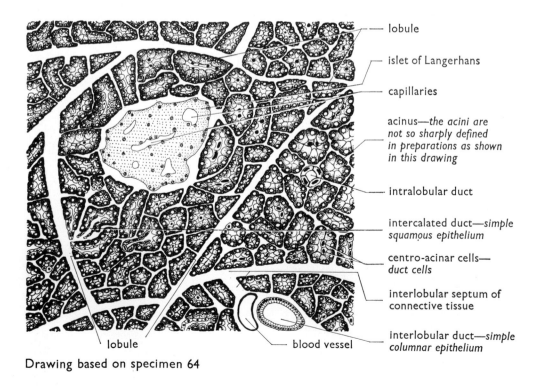

lobule

islet of Langerhans

capillaries

acinus—*the acini are
not so sharply defined
in preparations as shown
in this drawing*

intralobular duct

intercalated duct—*simple
squamous epithelium*

centro-acinar cells—
duct cells

interlobular septum of
connective tissue

interlobular duct—*simple
columnar epithelium*

lobule

blood vessel

Drawing based on specimen 64

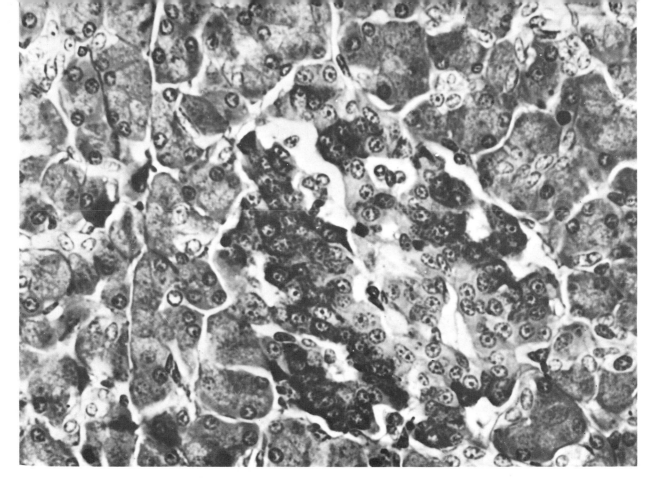

65. Islet of Langerhans, T.S. (sheep), mag. 575×

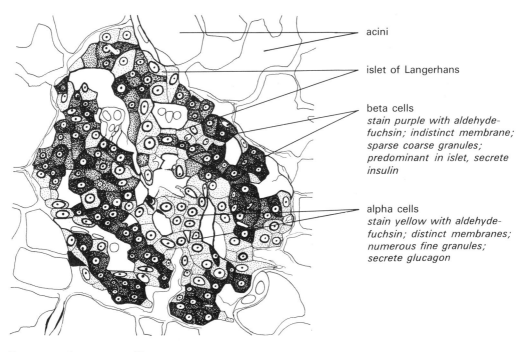

acini

islet of Langerhans

beta cells
stain purple with aldehyde-fuchsin; indistinct membrane; sparse coarse granules; predominant in islet, secrete insulin

alpha cells
stain yellow with aldehyde-fuchsin; distinct membranes; numerous fine granules; secrete glucagon

Drawing of specimen 65

THE UROGENITAL SYSTEM

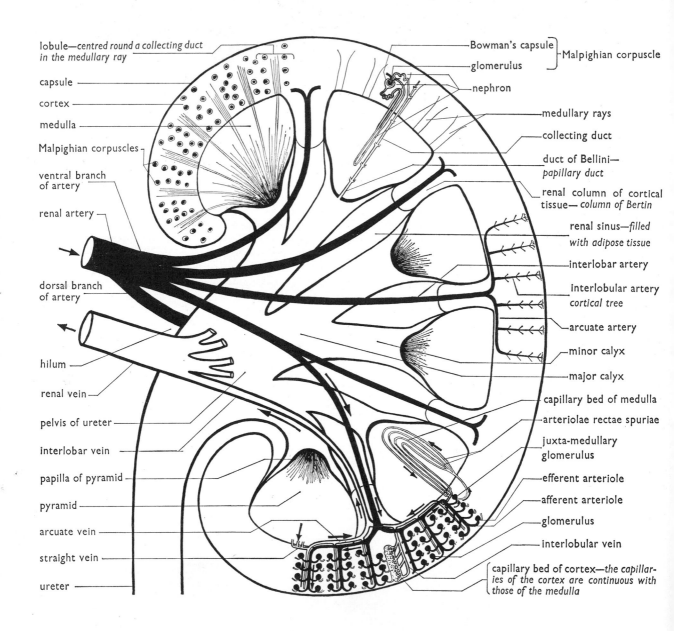

lobule—*centred round a collecting duct in the medullary ray*

capsule

cortex

medulla

Malpighian corpuscles

ventral branch of artery

renal artery

dorsal branch of artery

hilum

renal vein

pelvis of ureter

interlobar vein

papilla of pyramid

pyramid

arcuate vein

straight vein

ureter

Bowman's capsule ⎤
glomerulus ⎦ Malpighian corpuscle

nephron

medullary rays

collecting duct

duct of Bellini—*papillary duct*

renal column of cortical tissue—*column of Bertin*

renal sinus—*filled with adipose tissue*

interlobar artery

interlobular artery *cortical tree*

arcuate artery

minor calyx

major calyx

capillary bed of medulla

arteriolae rectae spuriae

juxta-medullary glomerulus

efferent arteriole

afferent arteriole

glomerulus

interlobular vein

capillary bed of cortex—*the capillaries of the cortex are continuous with those of the medulla*

DIAGRAM OF STRUCTURE OF KIDNEY

82

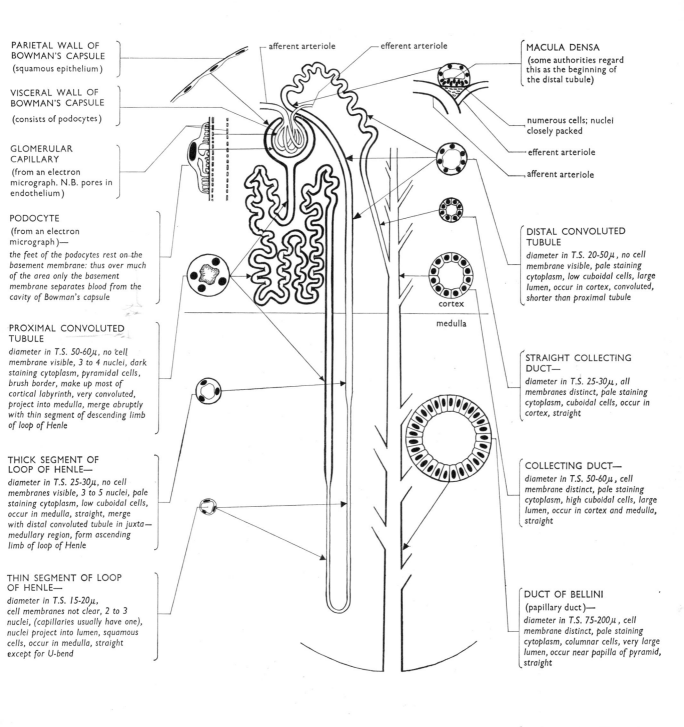

PARIETAL WALL OF BOWMAN'S CAPSULE
(squamous epithelium)

VISCERAL WALL OF BOWMAN'S CAPSULE
(consists of podocytes)

GLOMERULAR CAPILLARY
(from an electron micrograph. N.B. pores in endothelium)

PODOCYTE
(from an electron micrograph)—
the feet of the podocytes rest on the basement membrane: thus over much of the area only the basement membrane separates blood from the cavity of Bowman's capsule

PROXIMAL CONVOLUTED TUBULE
diameter in T.S. 50-60μ, no cell membrane visible, 3 to 4 nuclei, dark staining cytoplasm, pyramidal cells, brush border, make up most of cortical labyrinth, very convoluted, project into medulla, merge abruptly with thin segment of descending limb of loop of Henle

THICK SEGMENT OF LOOP OF HENLE—
diameter in T.S. 25-30μ, no cell membranes visible, 3 to 5 nuclei, pale staining cytoplasm, low cuboidal cells, occur in medulla, straight, merge with distal convoluted tubule in juxta—medullary region, form ascending limb of loop of Henle

THIN SEGMENT OF LOOP OF HENLE—
diameter in T.S. 15-20μ, cell membranes not clear, 2 to 3 nuclei, (capillaries usually have one), nuclei project into lumen, squamous cells, occur in medulla, straight except for U-bend

afferent arteriole

efferent arteriole

MACULA DENSA
(some authorities regard this as the beginning of the distal tubule)

numerous cells; nuclei closely packed

efferent arteriole

afferent arteriole

DISTAL CONVOLUTED TUBULE
diameter in T.S. 20-50μ, no cell membrane visible, pale staining cytoplasm, low cuboidal cells, large lumen, occur in cortex, convoluted, shorter than proximal tubule

cortex

medulla

STRAIGHT COLLECTING DUCT—
diameter in T.S. 25-30μ, all membranes distinct, pale staining cytoplasm, cuboidal cells, occur in cortex, straight

COLLECTING DUCT—
diameter in T.S. 50-60μ, cell membrane distinct, pale staining cytoplasm, high cuboidal cells, large lumen, occur in cortex and medulla, straight

DUCT OF BELLINI
(papillary duct)—
diameter in T.S. 75-200μ, cell membrane distinct, pale staining cytoplasm, columnar cells, very large lumen, occur near papilla of pyramid, straight

DIAGRAM OF NEPHRON

A nephron consists of Bowman's capsule, glomerulus, proximal convoluted tubule, loop of Henle and distal convoluted tubule.

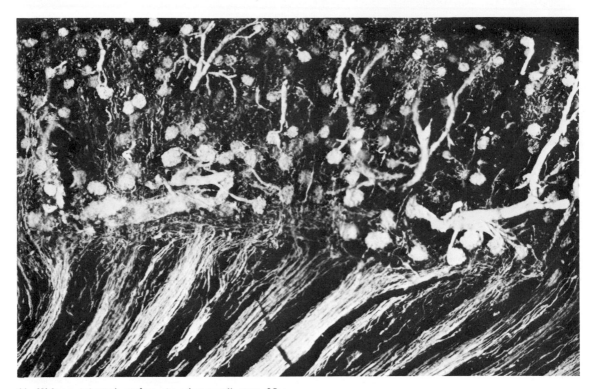

66. **Kidney,** injected, surface view (mammal), mag. 25 ×

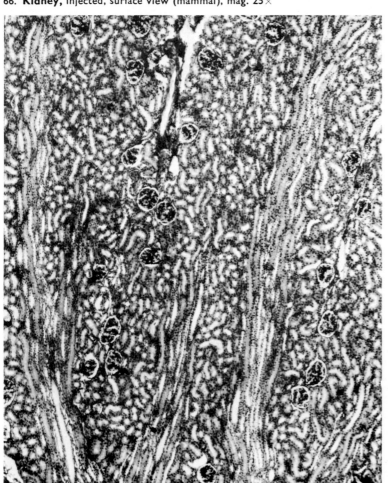

67. **Kidney,** cortex, L.S. (monkey), mag. 40

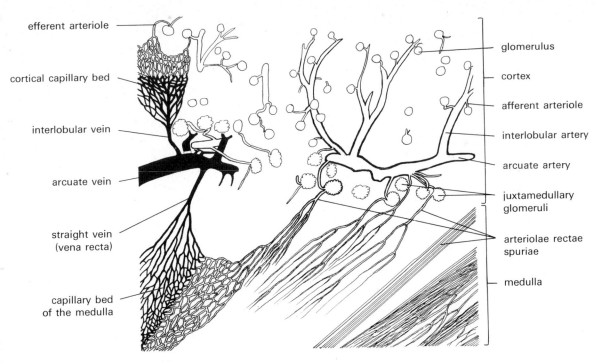

efferent arteriole

cortical capillary bed

interlobular vein

arcuate vein

straight vein
(vena recta)

capillary bed
of the medulla

glomerulus

cortex

afferent arteriole

interlobular artery

arcuate artery

juxtamedullary
glomeruli

arteriolae rectae
spuriae

medulla

Drawing based on specimen 66

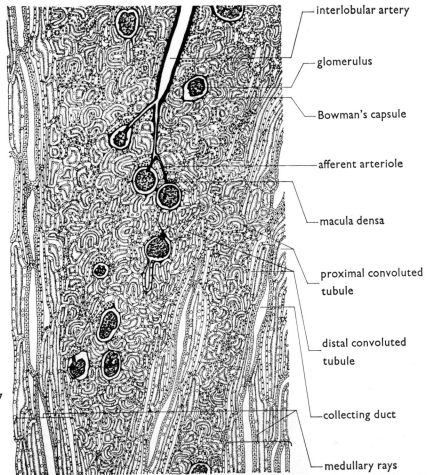

interlobular artery

glomerulus

Bowman's capsule

afferent arteriole

macula densa

proximal convoluted
tubule

distal convoluted
tubule

collecting duct

Drawing of specimen 67

medullary rays

85

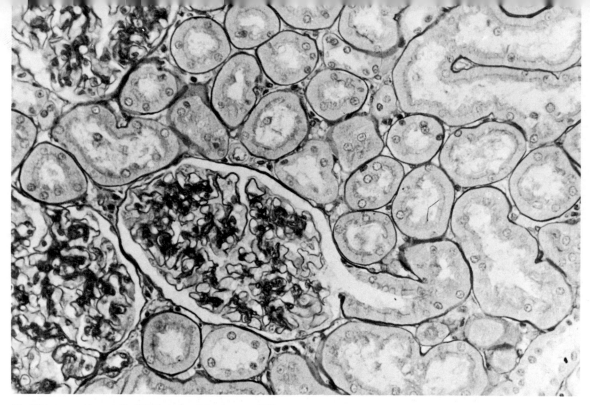

68. **Kidney,** cortex, L.S., P.A.S. stained (rat), mag. 575×

69. **Renal corpuscle,** L.S. (baboon), mag. 650×

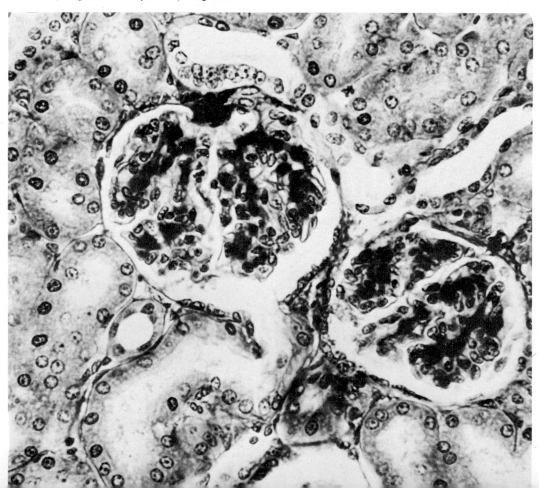

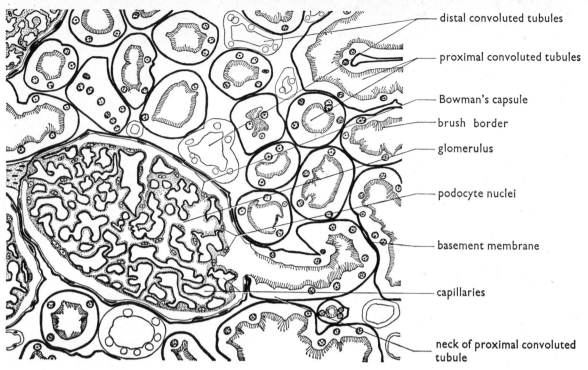

distal convoluted tubules

proximal convoluted tubules

Bowman's capsule

brush border

glomerulus

podocyte nuclei

basement membrane

capillaries

neck of proximal convoluted tubule

Drawing of specimen 68

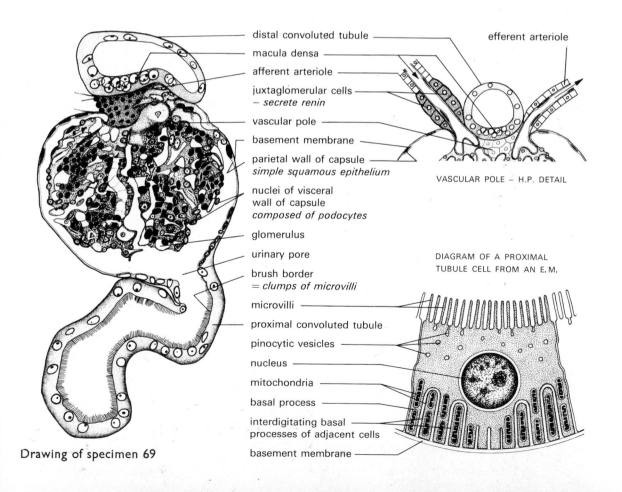

distal convoluted tubule

macula densa

afferent arteriole

juxtaglomerular cells
— *secrete renin*

vascular pole

basement membrane

parietal wall of capsule
simple squamous epithelium

nuclei of visceral
wall of capsule
composed of podocytes

glomerulus

urinary pore

brush border
= *clumps of microvilli*

microvilli

proximal convoluted tubule

pinocytic vesicles

nucleus

mitochondria

basal process

interdigitating basal
processes of adjacent cells

basement membrane

efferent arteriole

VASCULAR POLE – H.P. DETAIL

DIAGRAM OF A PROXIMAL
TUBULE CELL FROM AN E.M.

Drawing of specimen 69

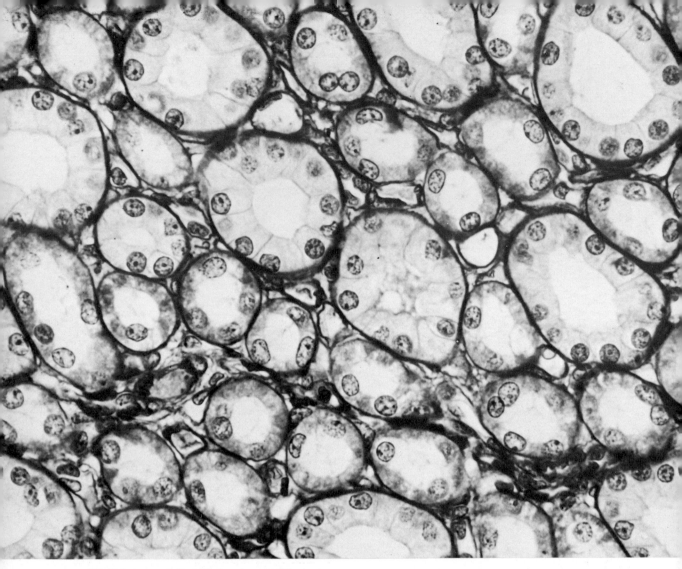

70. **Kidney,** medulla, T.S. (man), mag. 850×

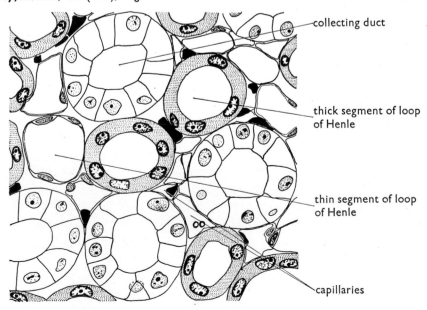

collecting duct

thick segment of loop
of Henle

thin segment of loop
of Henle

capillaries

Drawing based on specimen 70

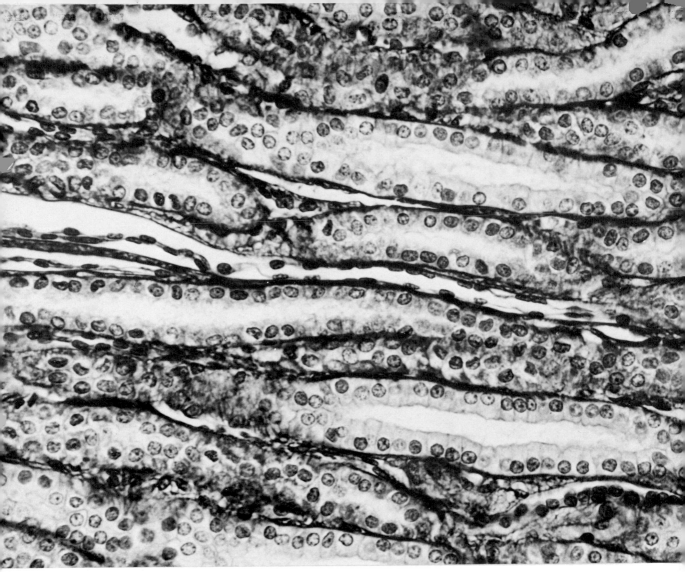

71. **Kidney,** medulla, L.S. (man), mag. 750×

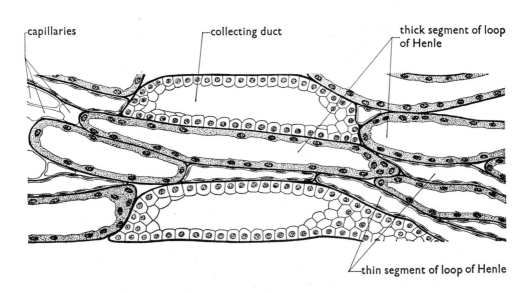

capillaries   collecting duct   thick segment of loop of Henle

thin segment of loop of Henle

Drawing based on specimen 71

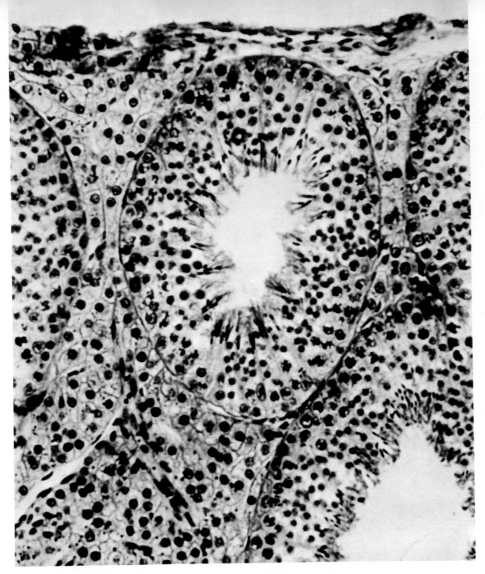

72. **Testis**, T.S. (cat), mag. 400×

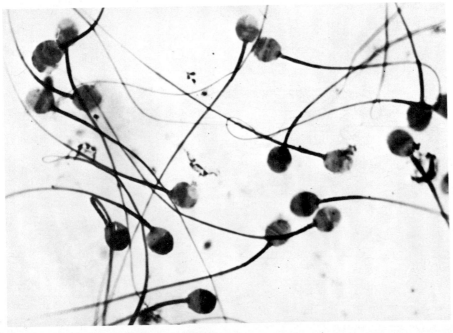

73. **Spermatozoa**, E. (mamm

mag. 1800×

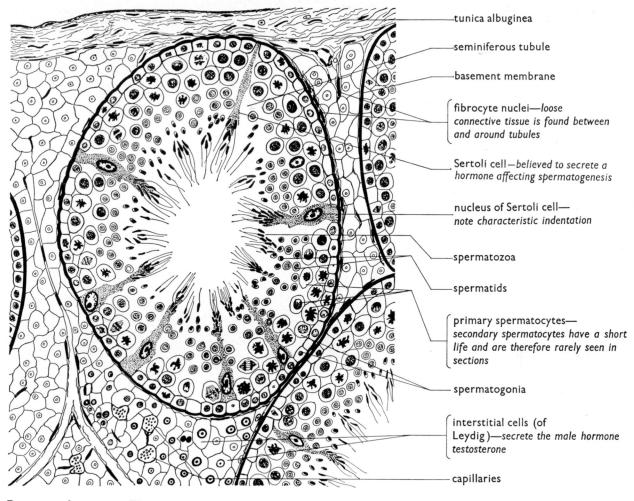

tunica albuginea

seminiferous tubule

basement membrane

fibrocyte nuclei—*loose connective tissue is found between and around tubules*

Sertoli cell—*believed to secrete a hormone affecting spermatogenesis*

nucleus of Sertoli cell— *note characteristic indentation*

spermatozoa

spermatids

primary spermatocytes— *secondary spermatocytes have a short life and are therefore rarely seen in sections*

spermatogonia

interstitial cells (of Leydig)—*secrete the male hormone testosterone*

capillaries

Drawing of specimen 72

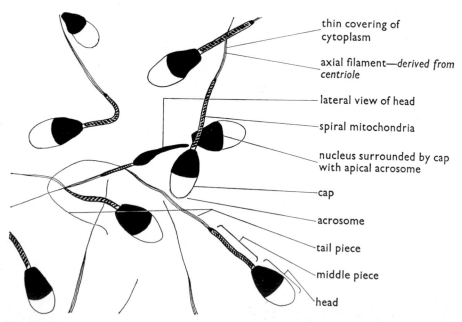

thin covering of cytoplasm

axial filament—*derived from centriole*

lateral view of head

spiral mitochondria

nucleus surrounded by cap with apical acrosome

cap

acrosome

tail piece

middle piece

head

Drawing based on specimen 73

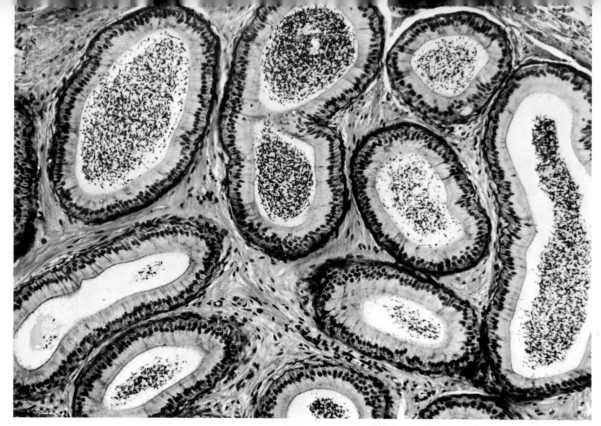

74. **Epididymis,** T.S. (cat), mag. 400 ×

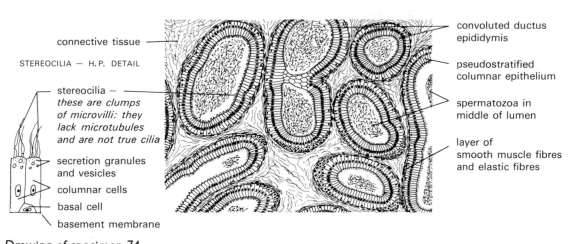

connective tissue

STEREOCILIA — H.P. DETAIL

stereocilia —
*these are clumps
of microvilli: they
lack microtubules
and are not true cilia*

secretion granules
and vesicles

columnar cells

basal cell

basement membrane

convoluted ductus
epididymis

pseudostratified
columnar epithelium

spermatozoa in
middle of lumen

layer of
smooth muscle fibres
and elastic fibres

Drawing of specimen 74

75. **Epididymis,** T.S., stereocilia (mammal), mag. 850 ×

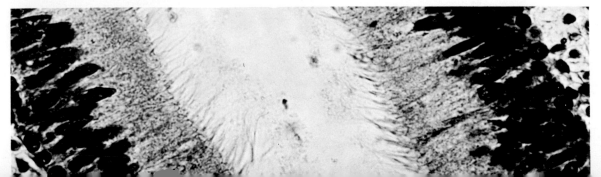

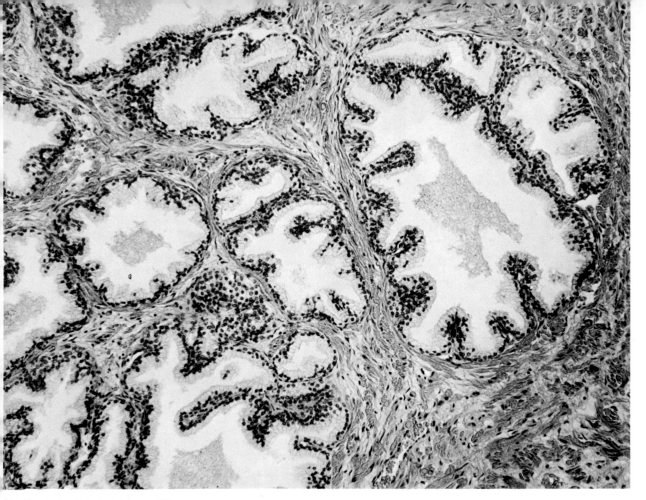

76. Prostate, T.S. (man), mag. 450 ×

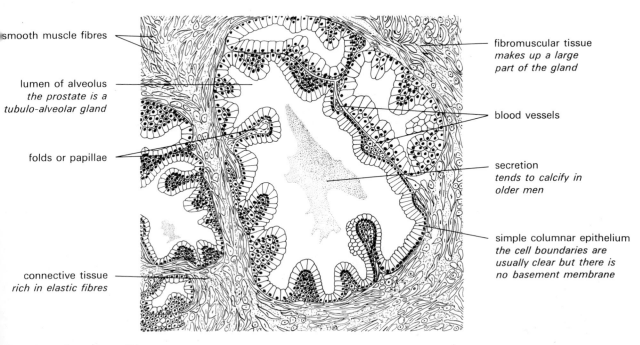

smooth muscle fibres

lumen of alveolus
*the prostate is a
tubulo-alveolar gland*

folds or papillae

connective tissue
rich in elastic fibres

fibromuscular tissue
*makes up a large
part of the gland*

blood vessels

secretion
*tends to calcify in
older men*

simple columnar epithelium
*the cell boundaries are
usually clear but there is
no basement membrane*

Drawing of specimen 76

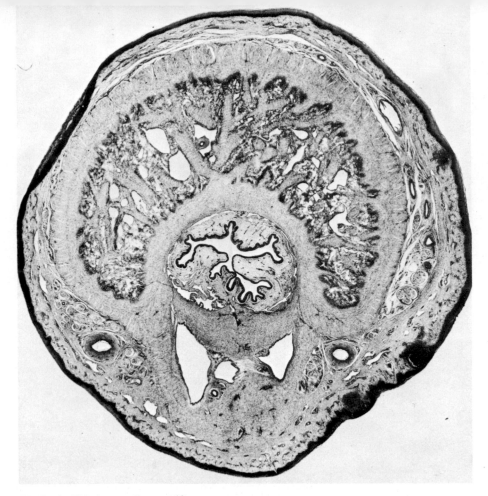

77. Penis, T.S. (mammal), mag. 10×

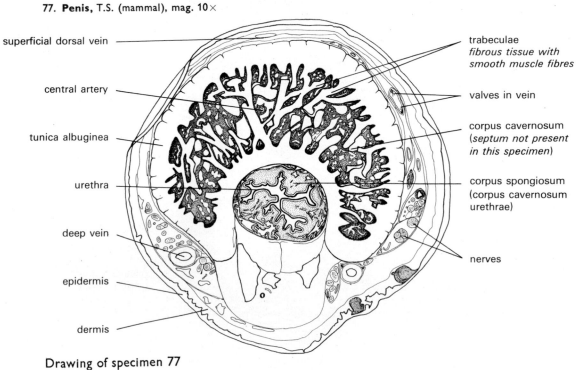

superficial dorsal vein

central artery

tunica albuginea

urethra

deep vein

epidermis

dermis

trabeculae
*fibrous tissue with
smooth muscle fibres*

valves in vein

corpus cavernosum
(*septum not present
in this specimen*)

corpus spongiosum
(corpus cavernosum
urethrae)

nerves

Drawing of specimen 77

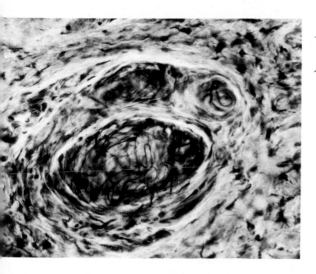

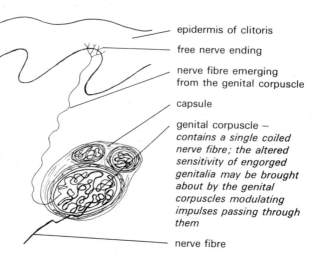

epidermis of clitoris

free nerve ending

nerve fibre emerging
from the genital corpuscle

capsule

genital corpuscle —
*contains a single coiled
nerve fibre; the altered
sensitivity of engorged
genitalia may be brought
about by the genital
corpuscles modulating
impulses passing through
them*

nerve fibre

Genital corpuscle, L.S. (mammalian clitoris, L.S.), mag. 900×

Drawing of specimen 78

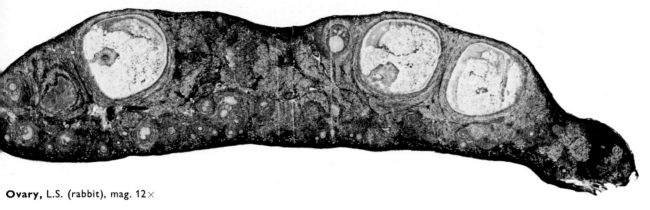

Ovary, L.S. (rabbit), mag. 12×

mature Graafian follicle — theca — cortex — medulla — stroma — germinal epithelium

secondary oocyte — tunica albuginea

mesovarium

blood vessels — developing follicles

Drawing of specimen 79

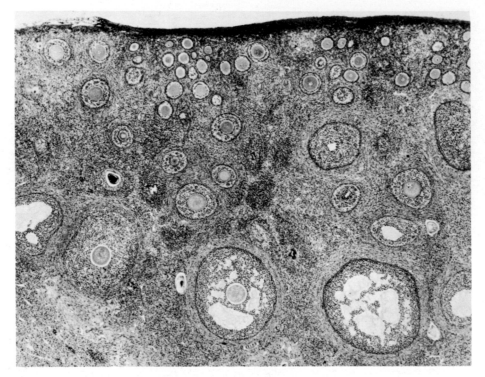

80. **Ovary,** developing follicles, L.S. (rabbit), mag. 175×

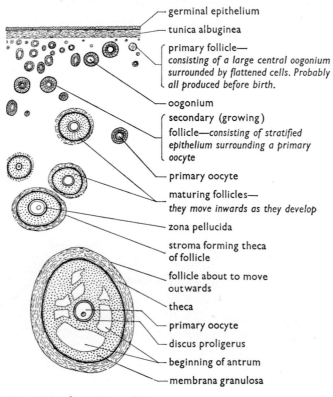

germinal epithelium

tunica albuginea

primary follicle—
*consisting of a large central oogonium
surrounded by flattened cells. Probably
all produced before birth.*

oogonium

secondary (growing)
follicle—*consisting of stratified
epithelium surrounding a primary
oocyte*

primary oocyte

maturing follicles—
they move inwards as they develop

zona pellucida

stroma forming theca
of follicle

follicle about to move
outwards

theca

primary oocyte

discus proligerus

beginning of antrum

membrana granulosa

Drawing of specimen 80

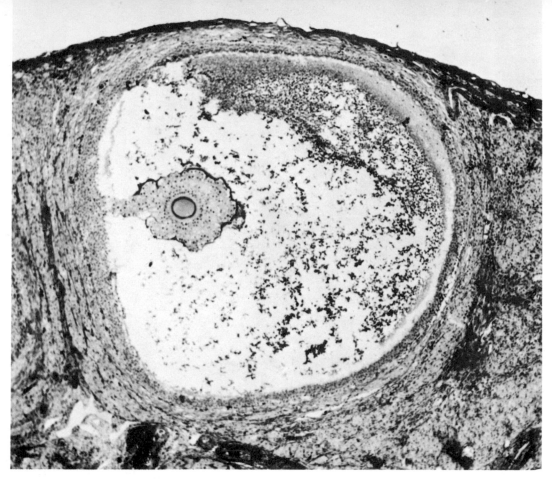

81. Graafian follicle, L.S. (rabbit), mag. 60 ×

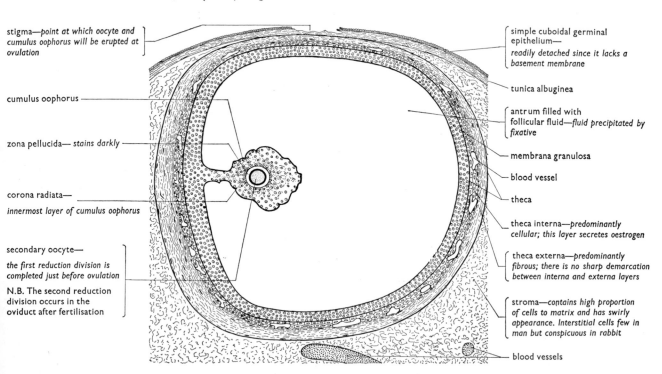

stigma—*point at which oocyte and cumulus oophorus will be erupted at ovulation*

cumulus oophorus

zona pellucida— *stains darkly*

corona radiata—

innermost layer of cumulus oophorus

secondary oocyte—

the first reduction division is completed just before ovulation

N.B. The second reduction division occurs in the oviduct after fertilisation

simple cuboidal germinal epithelium—

readily detached since it lacks a basement membrane

tunica albuginea

antrum filled with follicular fluid—*fluid precipitated by fixative*

membrana granulosa

blood vessel

theca

theca interna—*predominantly cellular; this layer secretes oestrogen*

theca externa—*predominantly fibrous; there is no sharp demarcation between interna and externa layers*

stroma—*contains high proportion of cells to matrix and has swirly appearance. Interstitial cells few in man but conspicuous in rabbit*

blood vessels

Drawing of specimen 81

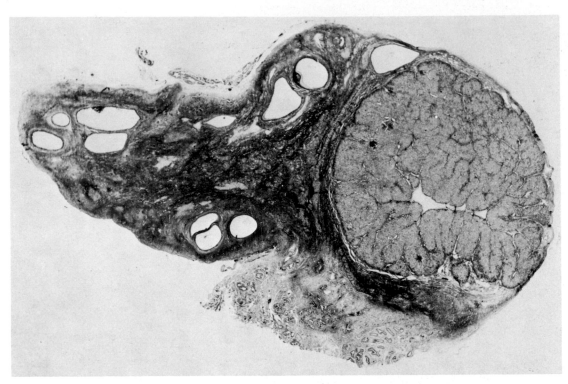

82. Corpus luteum, L.S. (human), mag. 3×

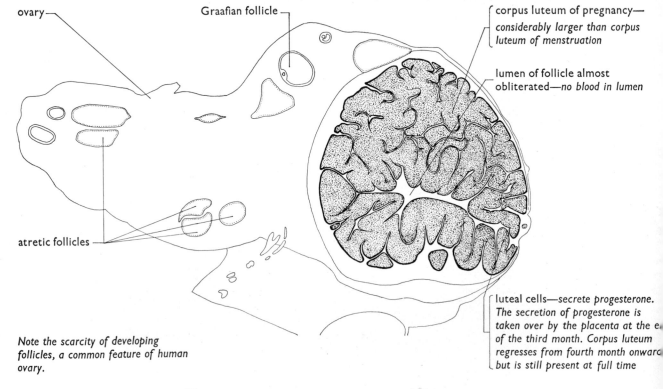

ovary

Graafian follicle

corpus luteum of pregnancy—*considerably larger than corpus luteum of menstruation*

lumen of follicle almost obliterated—*no blood in lumen*

atretic follicles

luteal cells—*secrete progesterone. The secretion of progesterone is taken over by the placenta at the e... of the third month. Corpus luteum regresses from fourth month onwar... but is still present at full time*

Note the scarcity of developing follicles, a common feature of human ovary.

Drawing of specimen 82

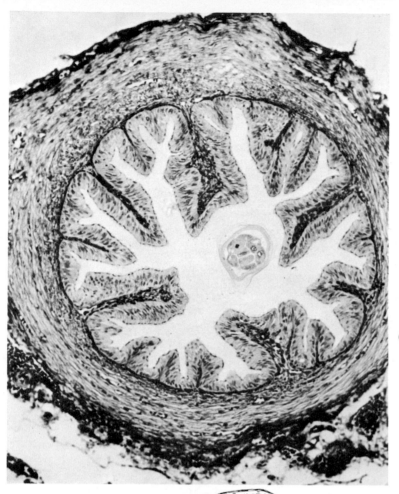

83. **Oviduct,** T.S., with developing morula, T.S. (rabbit), mag. 50×

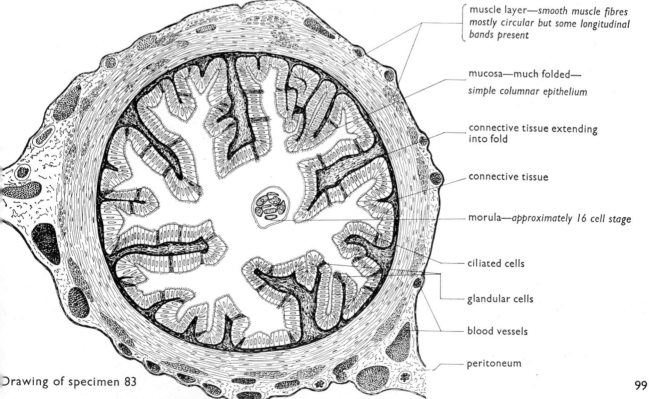

muscle layer—*smooth muscle fibres mostly circular but some longitudinal bands present*

mucosa—much folded—
simple columnar epithelium

connective tissue extending into fold

connective tissue

morula—*approximately 16 cell stage*

ciliated cells

glandular cells

blood vessels

peritoneum

Drawing of specimen 83

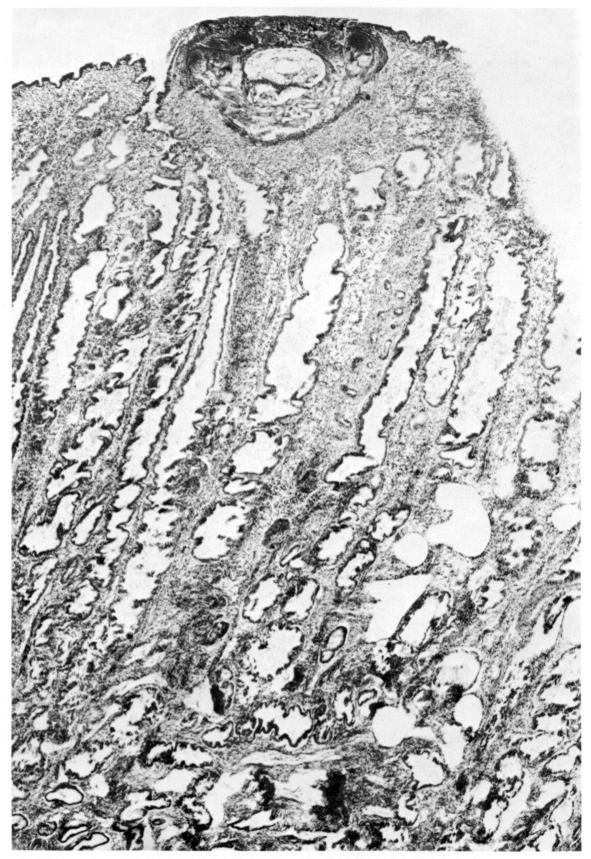

84. **Uterus,** pregnant with ovum, V.S. (human), mag. 25×

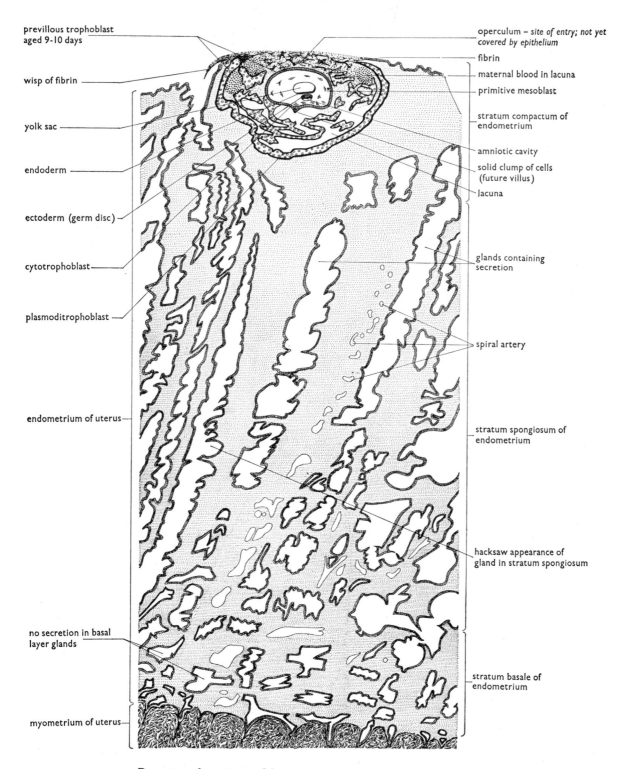

previllous trophoblast aged 9-10 days

wisp of fibrin

yolk sac

endoderm

ectoderm (germ disc)

cytotrophoblast

plasmoditrophoblast

endometrium of uterus

no secretion in basal layer glands

myometrium of uterus

operculum = *site of entry; not yet covered by epithelium*

fibrin

maternal blood in lacuna

primitive mesoblast

stratum compactum of endometrium

amniotic cavity

solid clump of cells (future villus)

lacuna

glands containing secretion

spiral artery

stratum spongiosum of endometrium

hacksaw appearance of gland in stratum spongiosum

stratum basale of endometrium

Drawing of specimen 84

Follicular phase
day 5 to day 15 proliferation

endometrium grows to a thickness of 0.5 mm.

OVULATION

DAY 14 (±1 DAY)

endometrium
myometrium
only part of it is shown

stratum compactum
stratum spongiosum
stratum basale

Progestational phase
day 16 to day 27 secretion

endometrium grows to a thickness of 5.0 mm. or more

MENSTRUAL FLOW

SHOULD FERTILISATION OCCUR IMPLANTATION OF BLASTOCYST IS APPROXIMATELY BETWEEN DAY 20 & DAY 23

disrupted epithelium reforms; glands proliferate

Menstruation day 1 to day 4

stratum compactum & stratum spongiosum shed into lumen together with about 50 c.cs of blood

BEGINNING OF CYCLE
first discharge of blood

Ischaemia day 28

vasoconstriction of spiral artery; necrosis of stratum compactum

spiral artery

dilated gland showing "hacksaw" appearance

the secretion contains mucin and glycogen

EACH MENSTRUAL CYCLE STARTS APPROXIMATELY 14 DAYS AFTER OVULATION. MENSTRUAL PERIODS STOP DURING PREGNANCY

DIAGRAM OF THE CHANGES IN THE ENDOMETRIUM DURING A 28 DAY MENSTRUAL CYCLE

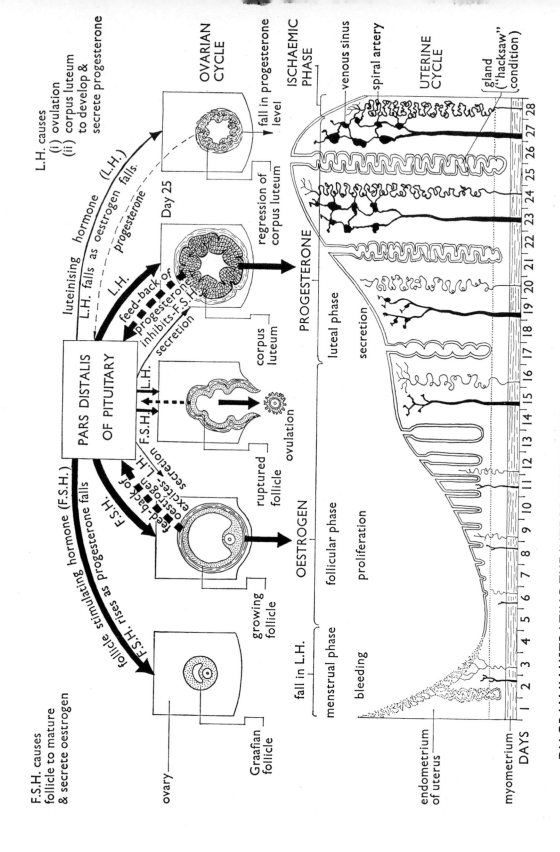

F.S.H. causes follicle to mature & secrete oestrogen

L.H. causes
(i) ovulation
(ii) corpus luteum to develop & secrete progesterone

OVARIAN CYCLE

luteinising hormone (L.H.)

L.H. falls as oestrogen falls.

L.H.

progesterone

feed-back of progesterone inhibits F.S.H. secretion

PARS DISTALIS OF PITUITARY

Day 25

fall in progesterone level

ISCHAEMIC PHASE

venous sinus

spiral artery

UTERINE CYCLE

gland ("hacksaw" condition)

regression of corpus luteum

PROGESTERONE

corpus luteum

luteal phase

secretion

F.S.H.

L.H.

feed-back of oestrogen excites L.H. secretion

ovulation

ruptured follicle

OESTROGEN

follicular phase

proliferation

follicle stimulating hormone (F.S.H.)

F.S.H. rises as progesterone falls

growing follicle

fall in L.H.

menstrual phase

bleeding

Graafian follicle

ovary

endometrium of uterus

myometrium

DAYS 1 2 3 4 5 6 7 8 9 10 11 12 13 14 15 16 17 18 19 20 21 22 23 24 25 26 27 28

DIAGRAM ILLUSTRATING THE INTEGRATION OF THE OVARIAN AND UTERINE CYCLES BY HORMONES

103

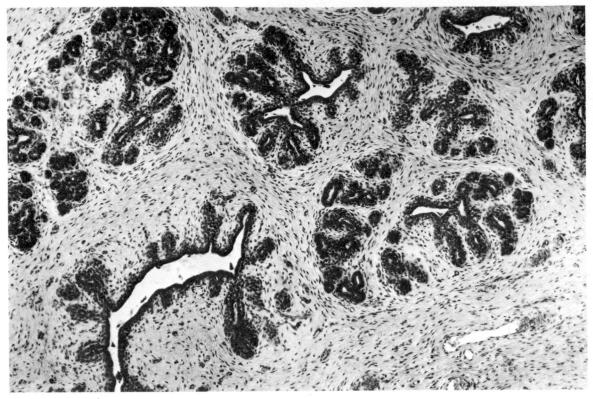

85. **Mammary gland,** inactive, T.S. (mammal), mag. 420×

lobules

intralobular connective
tissue
— *derived from the papillary
layer of the dermis; cellular
nature indicated by the
many nuclei*

interlobular connective
tissue
— *derived from the reticular
layer of the dermis;
coarse and relatively non-
cellular*

intralobular duct
— *branching repeatedly
within a lobule*

stratified columnar
epithelium of duct wall
— *composed of two
layers of cells*

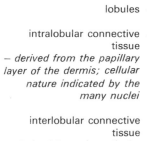
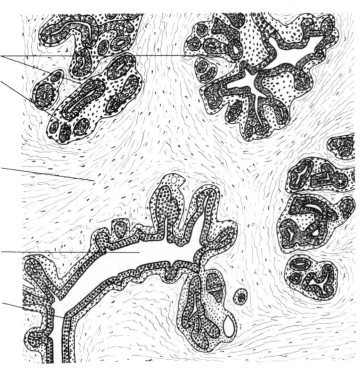

Drawing of specimen 85

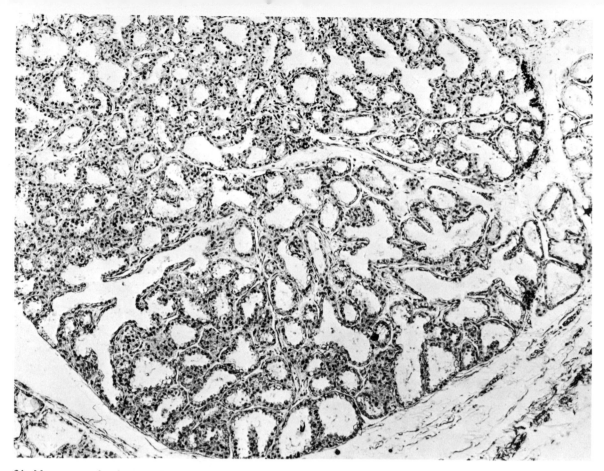

86. **Mammary gland,** active, T.S. (mammal), mag. 420×

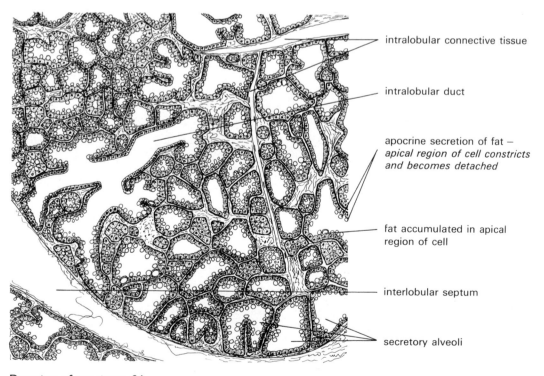

intralobular connective tissue

intralobular duct

apocrine secretion of fat –
*apical region of cell constricts
and becomes detached*

fat accumulated in apical
region of cell

interlobular septum

secretory alveoli

Drawing of specimen 86

THE SKIN

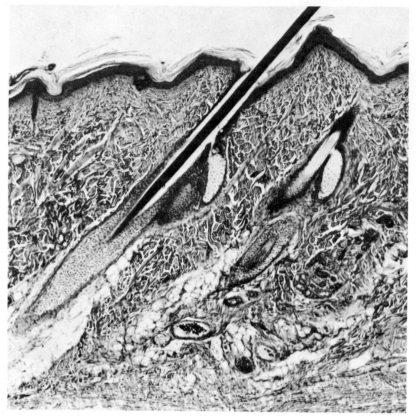

87. **Skin,** hairy, V.S. (baboon), mag. 50 ×

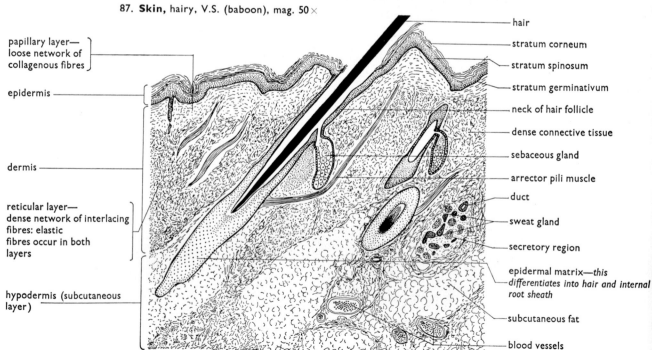

papillary layer—
loose network of
collagenous fibres

epidermis

dermis

reticular layer—
dense network of interlacing
fibres: elastic
fibres occur in both
layers

hypodermis (subcutaneous
layer)

hair

stratum corneum

stratum spinosum

stratum germinativum

neck of hair follicle

dense connective tissue

sebaceous gland

arrector pili muscle

duct

sweat gland

secretory region

epidermal matrix—*this
differentiates into hair and internal
root sheath*

subcutaneous fat

blood vessels

Drawing of specimen 87

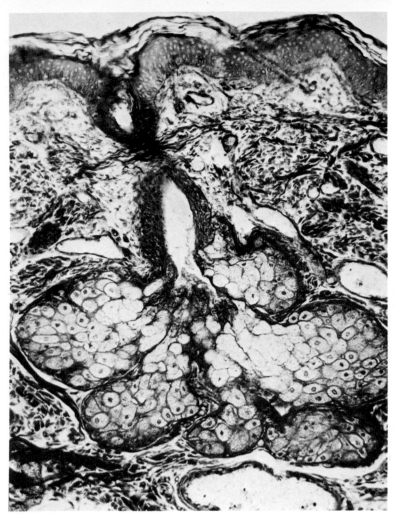

88. **Skin,** sebaceous gland detail, V.S. (baboon), mag. 10×

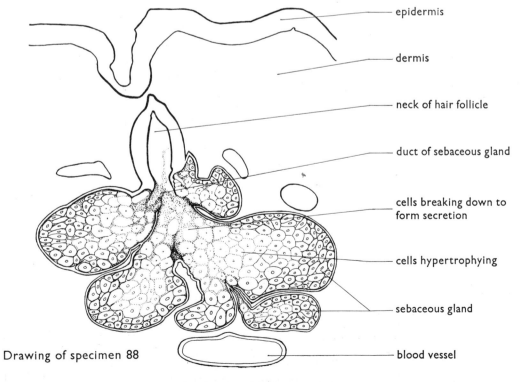

epidermis

dermis

neck of hair follicle

duct of sebaceous gland

cells breaking down to form secretion

cells hypertrophying

sebaceous gland

blood vessel

Drawing of specimen 88

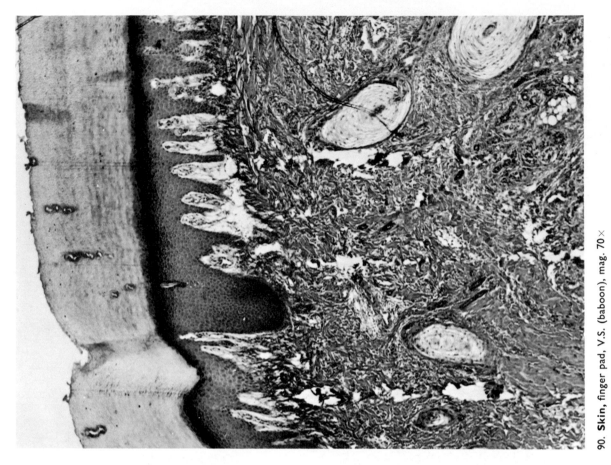

90. **Skin**, finger pad, V.S. (baboon), mag. 70 ×

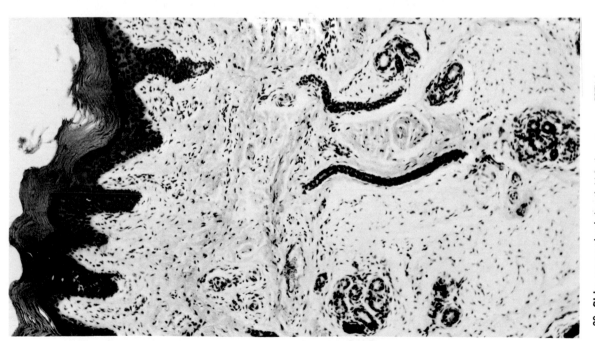

89. **Skin**, sweat gland detail, V.S. (man), mag. 135 ×

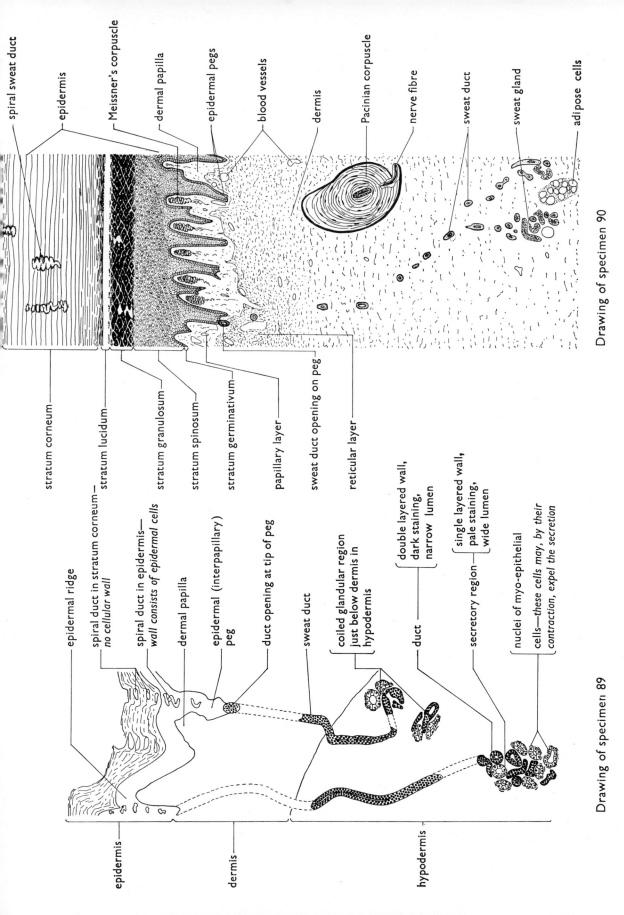

spiral sweat duct

epidermis

Meissner's corpuscle

dermal papilla

epidermal pegs

blood vessels

dermis

Pacinian corpuscle

nerve fibre

sweat duct

sweat gland

adipose cells

Drawing of specimen 90

stratum corneum

spiral duct in stratum corneum—*no cellular wall*

stratum lucidum

spiral duct in epidermis—*wall consists of epidermal cells*

stratum granulosum

stratum spinosum

stratum germinativum

papillary layer

sweat duct opening on peg

reticular layer

epidermal ridge

dermal papilla

epidermal (interpapillary) peg

duct opening at tip of peg

sweat duct

coiled glandular region just below dermis in hypodermis

double layered wall, dark staining, narrow lumen

duct

single layered wall, pale staining, wide lumen

secretory region

nuclei of myo-epithelial cells—*these cells may, by their contraction, expel the secretion*

epidermis

dermis

hypodermis

Drawing of specimen 89

109

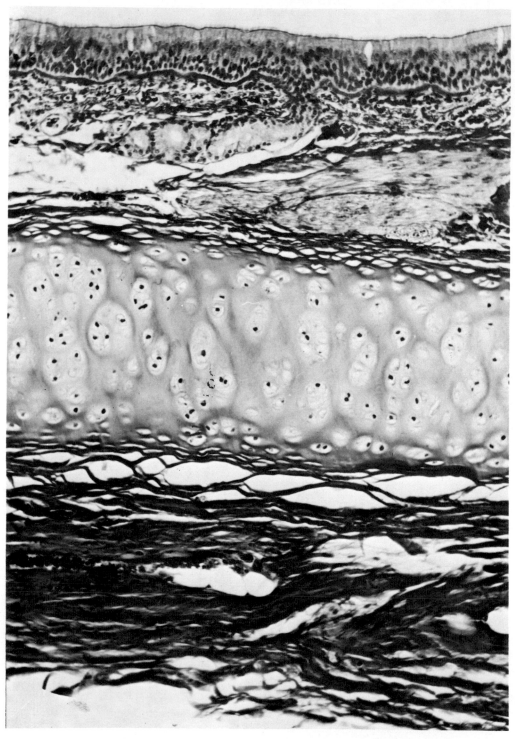

91. **Trachea**, T.S. (man), mag. 175×

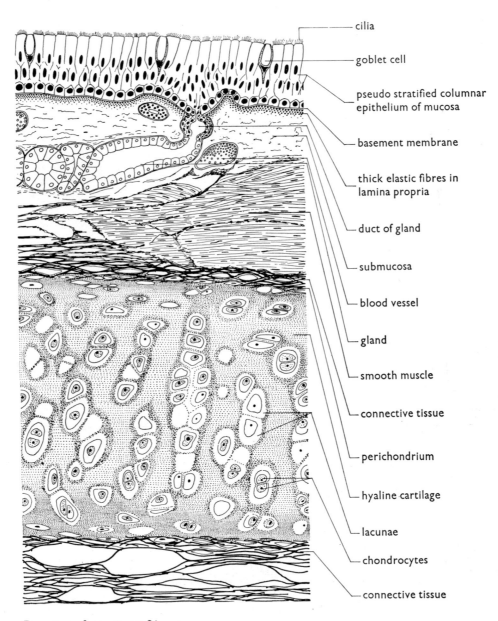

- cilia
- goblet cell
- pseudo stratified columnar epithelium of mucosa
- basement membrane
- thick elastic fibres in lamina propria
- duct of gland
- submucosa
- blood vessel
- gland
- smooth muscle
- connective tissue
- perichondrium
- hyaline cartilage
- lacunae
- chondrocytes
- connective tissue

Drawing of specimen 91

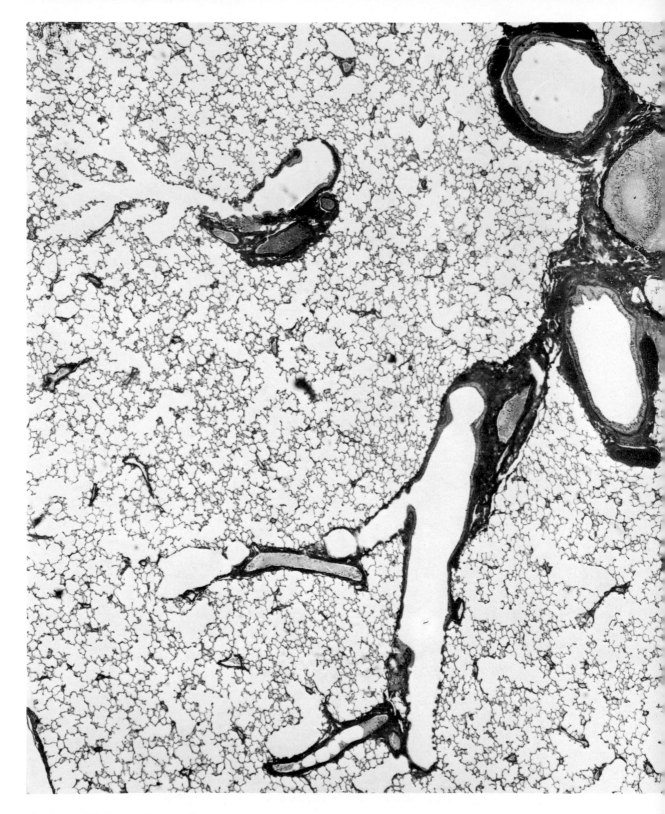

92. **Lung,** T.S. (mammal), mag. 40×

THE MAIN FEATURES OF THE LUNG

	Large bronchus	Small bronchus	Bronchiole	Terminal bronchiole	Respiratory bronchiole	Alveolar duct
Epithelium	pseudo-stratified, ciliated, columnar	pseudo-stratified, ciliated, columnar	pseudo-stratified, ciliated, columnar	simple ciliated columnar	simple cuboidal	simple cuboidal
Goblet cells	present	a few present	very scattered	absent	absent	absent
Cartilage	present	a little present	absent	absent	absent	absent
Glands	present	a few present	absent	absent	absent	absent
Smooth muscle	two sets—a right and a left— spiral	present	present	present	a few fibres present
Alveoli	absent	absent	absent	absent	present	prolific

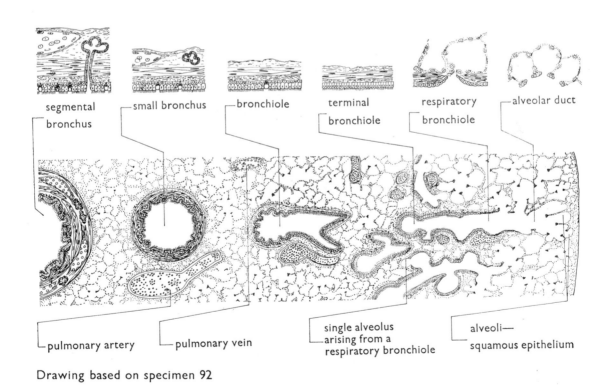

segmental bronchus   small bronchus   bronchiole   terminal bronchiole   respiratory bronchiole   alveolar duct

pulmonary artery   pulmonary vein   single alveolus arising from a respiratory bronchiole   alveoli— squamous epithelium

Drawing based on specimen 92

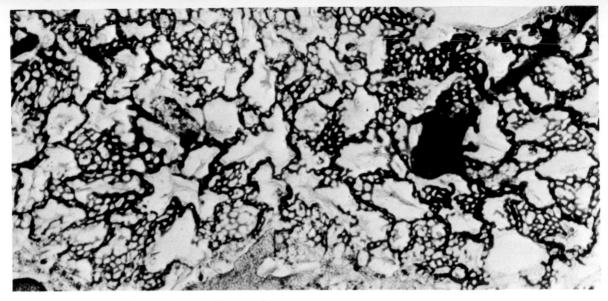

93. **Lung,** injected, T.S. (mammal), mag. 100×

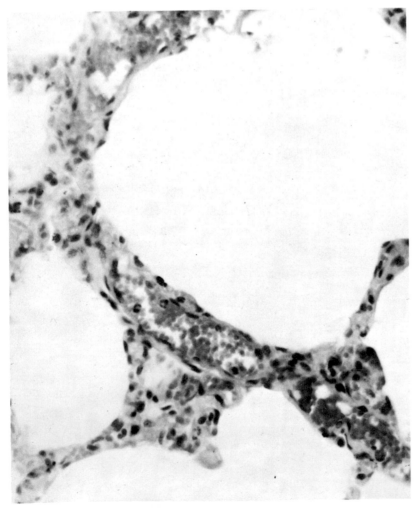

94. **Lung,** alveolar wall, T.S. (man), mag. 950×

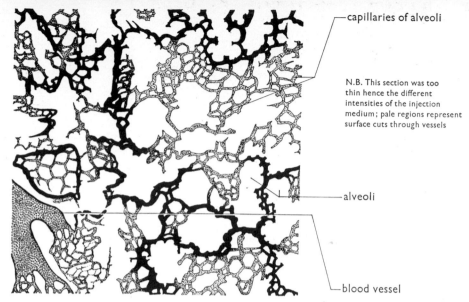

capillaries of alveoli

N.B. This section was too thin hence the different intensities of the injection medium; pale regions represent surface cuts through vessels

alveoli

blood vessel

Drawing based on specimen 93

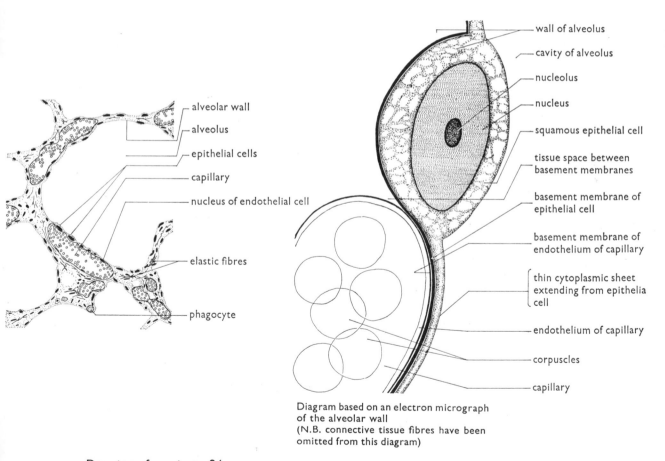

alveolar wall

alveolus

epithelial cells

capillary

nucleus of endothelial cell

elastic fibres

phagocyte

wall of alveolus

cavity of alveolus

nucleolus

nucleus

squamous epithelial cell

tissue space between basement membranes

basement membrane of epithelial cell

basement membrane of endothelium of capillary

thin cytoplasmic sheet extending from epithelial cell

endothelium of capillary

corpuscles

capillary

Diagram based on an electron micrograph of the alveolar wall
(N.B. connective tissue fibres have been omitted from this diagram)

Drawing of specimen 94

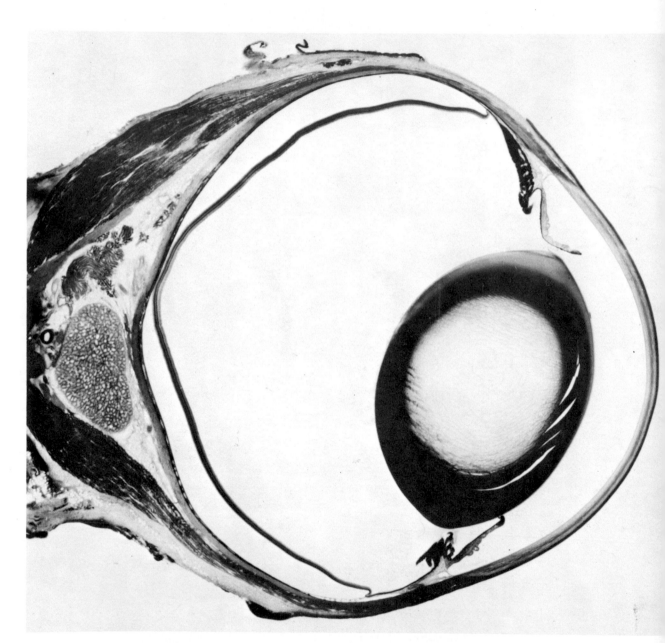

95. **Eye,** gross, T.S. (guinea pig), mag. 12×

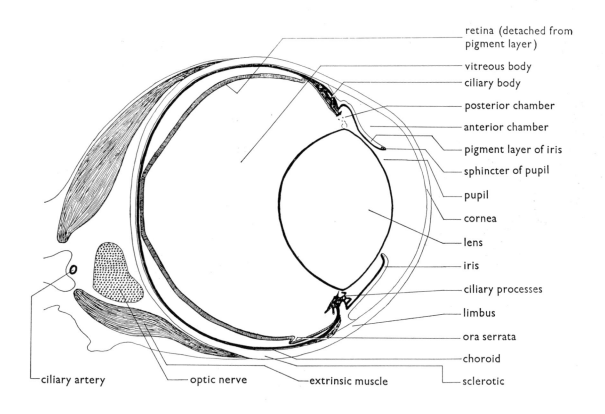

retina (detached from
pigment layer)

vitreous body

ciliary body

posterior chamber

anterior chamber

pigment layer of iris

sphincter of pupil

pupil

cornea

lens

iris

ciliary processes

limbus

ora serrata

choroid

sclerotic

ciliary artery

optic nerve

extrinsic muscle

Drawing of specimen 95

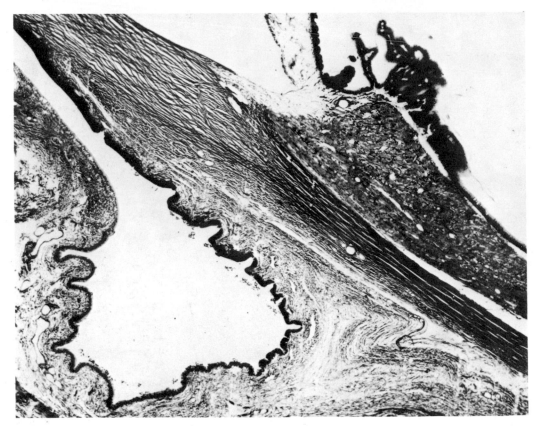

96. **Eye,** ciliary junction, T.S. (man), mag. 45 ×

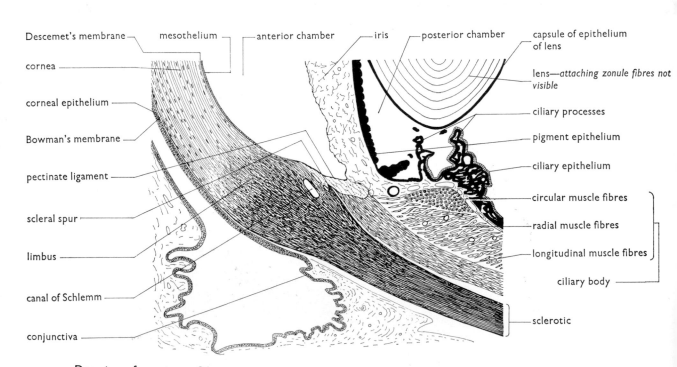

Descemet's membrane — mesothelium — anterior chamber — iris — posterior chamber — capsule of epithelium of lens

cornea

corneal epithelium

Bowman's membrane

pectinate ligament

scleral spur

limbus

canal of Schlemm

conjunctiva

lens—*attaching zonule fibres not visible*

ciliary processes

pigment epithelium

ciliary epithelium

circular muscle fibres

radial muscle fibres

longitudinal muscle fibres

ciliary body

sclerotic

Drawing of specimen 96

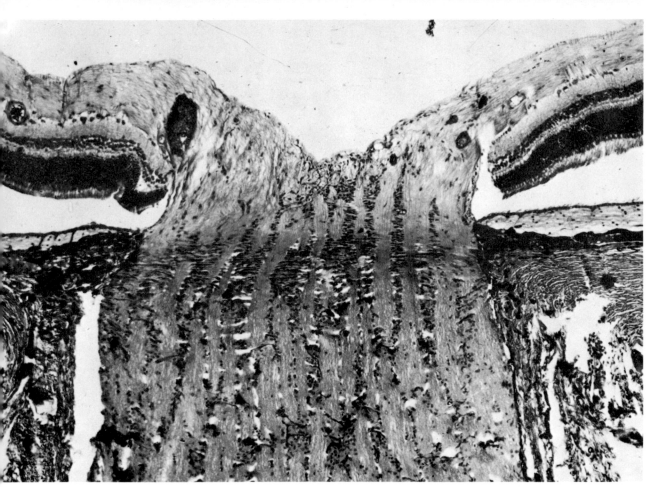

97. **Eye,** blind spot, T.S. (rabbit), mag. 50×

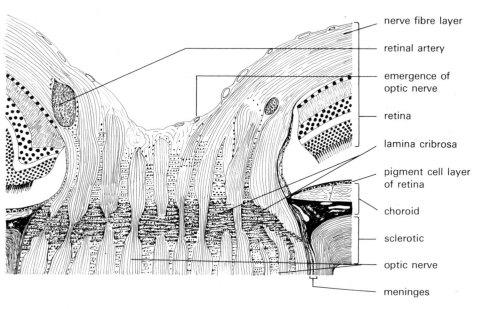

nerve fibre layer

retinal artery

emergence of
optic nerve

retina

lamina cribrosa

pigment cell layer
of retina

choroid

sclerotic

optic nerve

meninges

Drawing of specimen 97

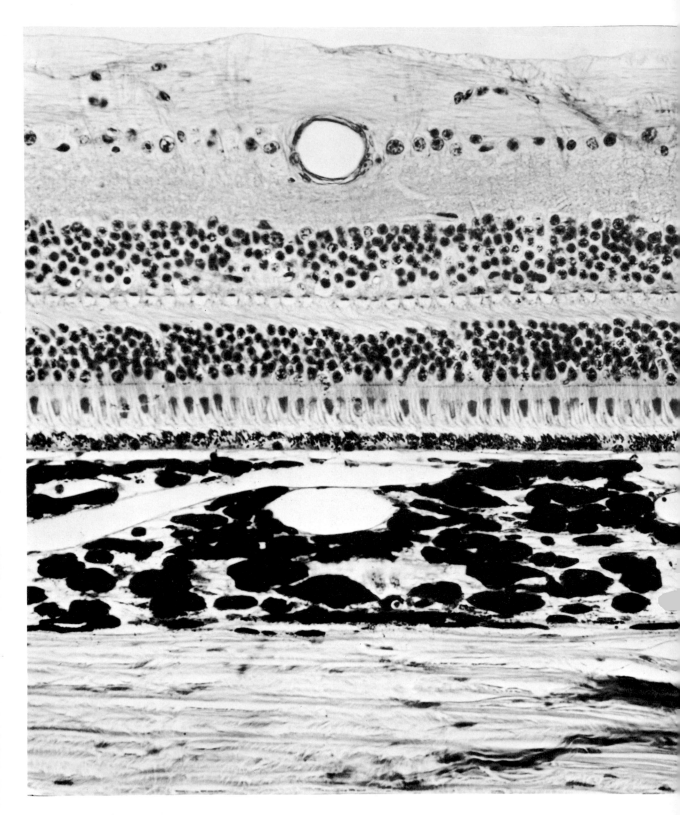

98. **Eye,** retina, V.S. (rabbit), mag. 1050×

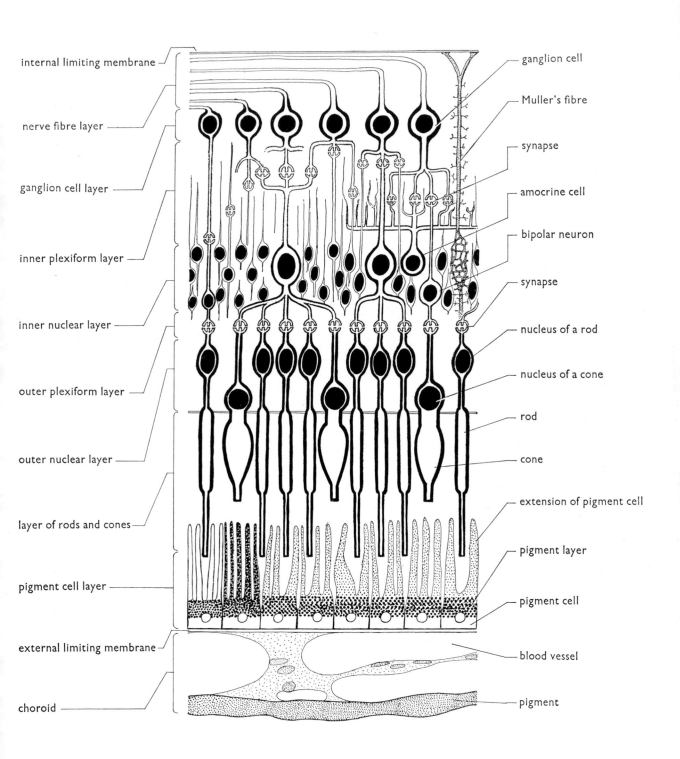

internal limiting membrane

nerve fibre layer

ganglion cell layer

inner plexiform layer

inner nuclear layer

outer plexiform layer

outer nuclear layer

layer of rods and cones

pigment cell layer

external limiting membrane

choroid

ganglion cell

Muller's fibre

synapse

amocrine cell

bipolar neuron

synapse

nucleus of a rod

nucleus of a cone

rod

cone

extension of pigment cell

pigment layer

pigment cell

blood vessel

pigment

Diagram to explain specimen 98

121

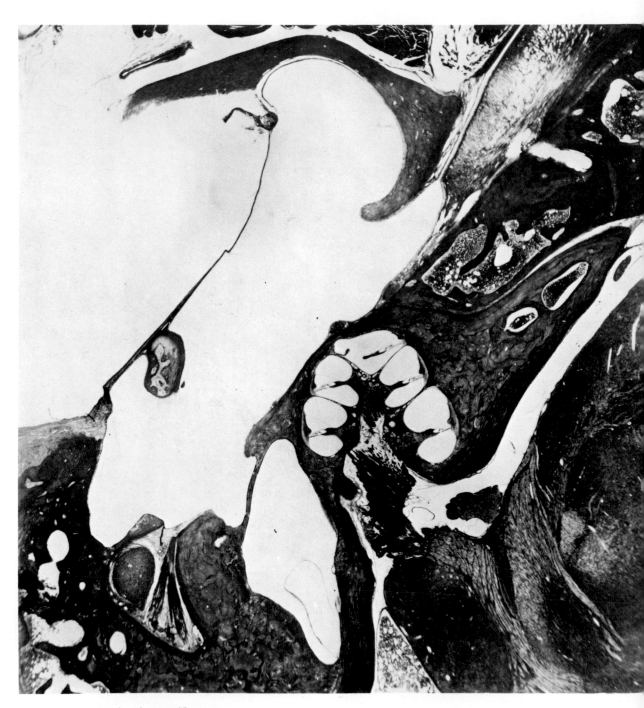

99. **Ear,** gross, H.S. (man), mag. 15×

front of head

temporal bone
epidermis
ciliated epithelium
external auditory meatus
helicotrema
spiral osseous lamina
tympanic cavity
modiolus
handle of malleus
cartilaginous perimeter of
stapedial base
fenestra vestibuli (ovalis)
vestibule
pyramid
tendon of stapedius muscle
facial (VIIth) nerve
stapedius muscle
temporal bone
mastoid air cells
macula
saccule
utricle

auditory (eustachian) tube
canal for tensor tympani
fissure
petrous temporal bone
cochlea
cochlear nerve
vestibular nerve
stato-acoustic (VIIIth)
nerve
temporal lobe of brain
cerebellum
choroid plexus

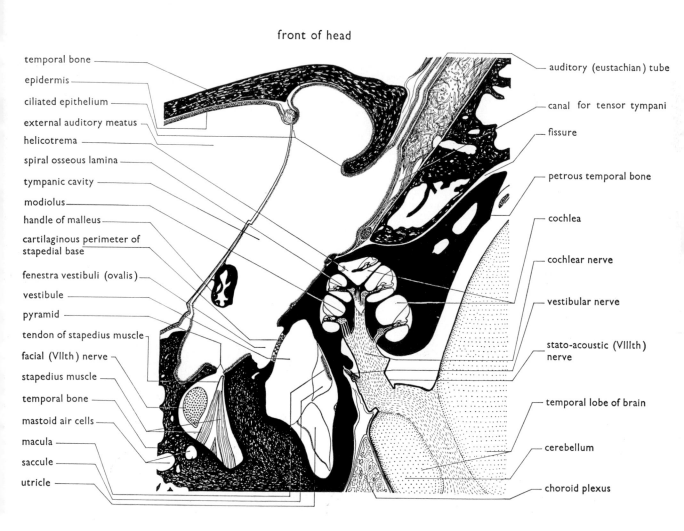

Drawing of specimen 99

123

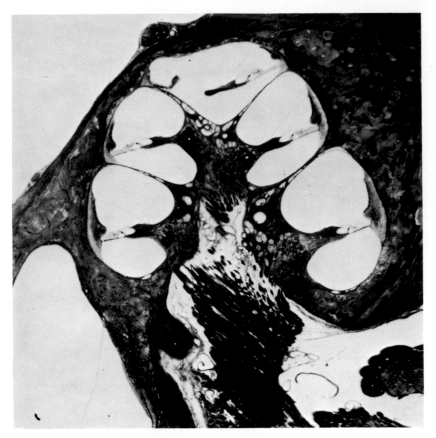

100. **Ear,** cochlea, H.S. (man), mag. 50×

101. **Ear,** organ of Corti, V.S. (man), mag. 175×

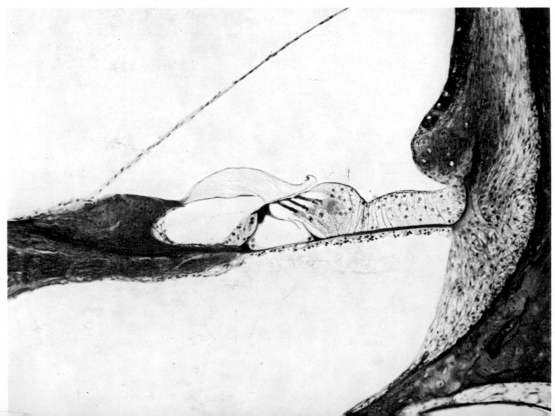

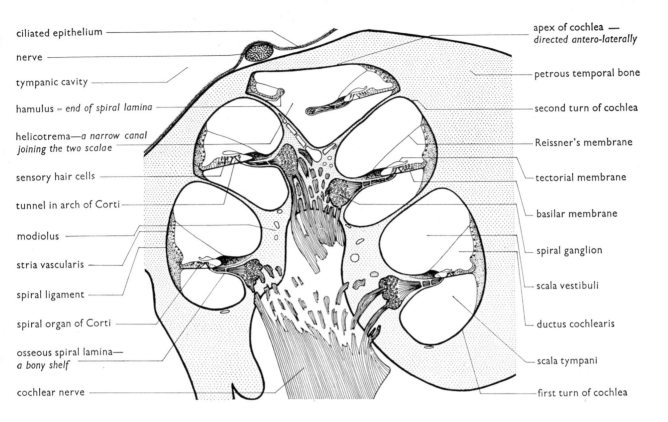

ciliated epithelium

nerve

tympanic cavity

hamulus = *end of spiral lamina*

helicotrema—*a narrow canal joining the two scalae*

sensory hair cells

tunnel in arch of Corti

modiolus

stria vascularis

spiral ligament

spiral organ of Corti

osseous spiral lamina— *a bony shelf*

cochlear nerve

apex of cochlea — *directed antero-laterally*

petrous temporal bone

second turn of cochlea

Reissner's membrane

tectorial membrane

basilar membrane

spiral ganglion

scala vestibuli

ductus cochlearis

scala tympani

first turn of cochlea

Drawing of specimen 100

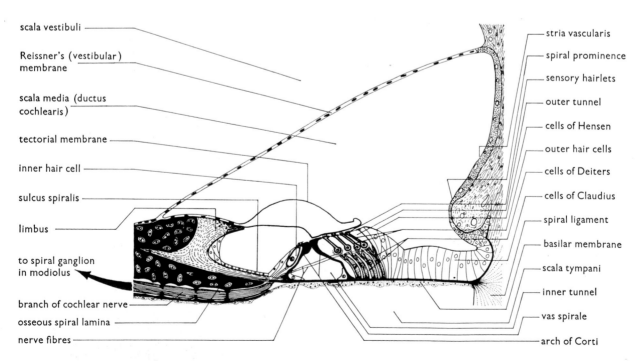

scala vestibuli

Reissner's (vestibular) membrane

scala media (ductus cochlearis)

tectorial membrane

inner hair cell

sulcus spiralis

limbus

to spiral ganglion in modiolus

branch of cochlear nerve

osseous spiral lamina

nerve fibres

stria vascularis

spiral prominence

sensory hairlets

outer tunnel

cells of Hensen

outer hair cells

cells of Deiters

cells of Claudius

spiral ligament

basilar membrane

scala tympani

inner tunnel

vas spirale

arch of Corti

Drawing of specimen 101

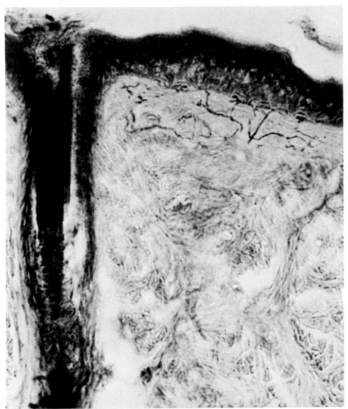

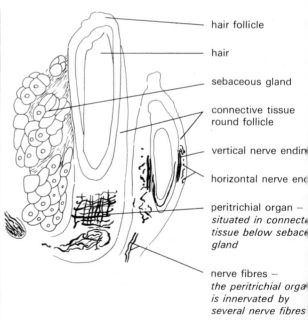

free nerve
endings

non-medullated
nerve fibre

medullated
nerve fibre

epiderm

dermis

Drawing of specimen 102

102. **Free nerve ending,** skin, V.S. (rabbit), mag. 150×

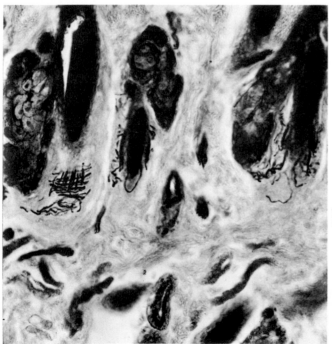

hair follicle

hair

sebaceous gland

connective tissue
round follicle

vertical nerve endin

horizontal nerve end

peritrichial organ —
*situated in connect.
tissue below sebac.
gland*

nerve fibres —
*the peritrichial orga
is innervated by
several nerve fibres*

Drawing of specimen 103

103. **Peritrichial nerve,** skin, V.S. (rabbit), mag. 150×

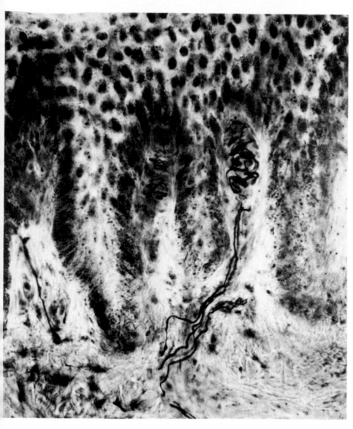

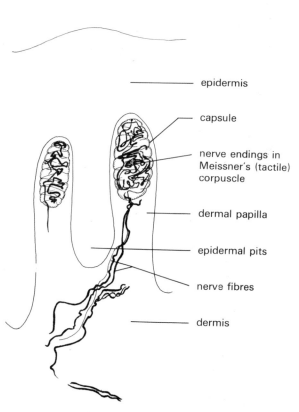

104. Meissner's corpuscle, skin, V.S. (baboon), mag. 575×

Drawing of specimen 104

- epidermis
- capsule
- nerve endings in Meissner's (tactile) corpuscle
- dermal papilla
- epidermal pits
- nerve fibres
- dermis

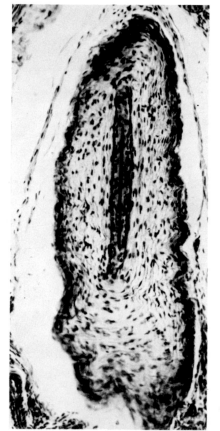

Pacinian corpuscle
capsule
outer zone
inner zone
non-medullated nerve fibre
medullated nerve fibre

terminal club-shaped processes *nerve impulses probably initiated here*

Drawing based on specimen 105

105. Pacinian corpuscle, pancreas, L.S. (cat), mag. 250×

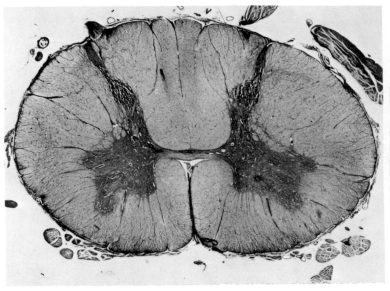

106. **Spinal cord,** cervical region, T.S. (man), mag. 7×

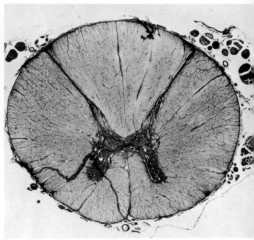

107. **Spinal cord,** thoracic region, T.S. (man), mag.

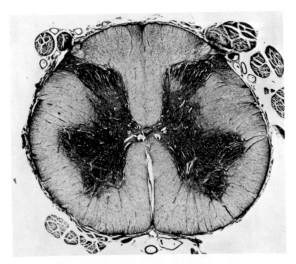

108. **Spinal cord,** lumbar region, T.S. (man), mag. 7×

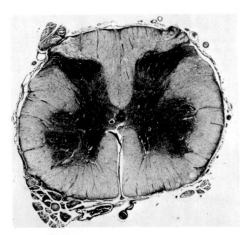

109. **Spinal cord,** sacral region, T.S. (man), mag. 7×

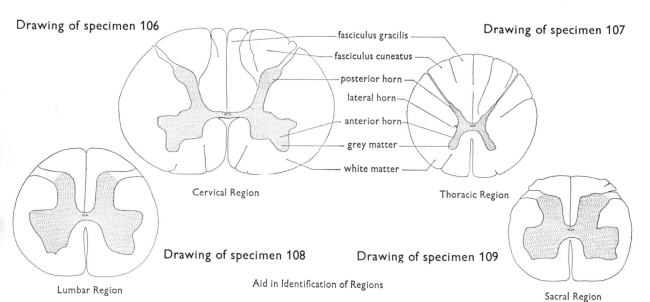

Drawing of specimen 106

fasciculus gracilis
fasciculus cuneatus
posterior horn
lateral horn
anterior horn
grey matter
white matter

Drawing of specimen 107

Cervical Region

Thoracic Region

Drawing of specimen 108

Drawing of specimen 109

Lumbar Region

Sacral Region

Aid in Identification of Regions

Region	Appearance in Cross Sections	White Matter	Grey Matter	Other Features
Cervical	large, oval	has greatest amount	posterior horns slender, anterior wide	fasciculus cuneatus as well as gracilis
Thoracic	small, round	considerable amount	posterior & anterior horns slender	lateral horn in some segments f. cuneatus in segments 1-4
Lumbar	larger than thoracic, anterior broader than posterior part	little	both horns wide	lateral horn in first two segments; fasciculus gracilis only
Sacral	small, slightly oval, almost surrounded by roots	very little	grey matter predominant; horns very wide	

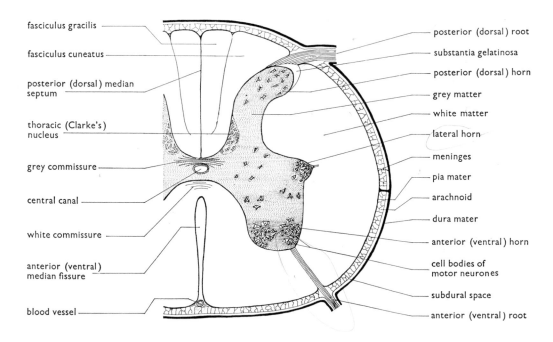

fasciculus gracilis
fasciculus cuneatus
posterior (dorsal) median septum
thoracic (Clarke's) nucleus
grey commissure
central canal
white commissure
anterior (ventral) median fissure
blood vessel

posterior (dorsal) root
substantia gelatinosa
posterior (dorsal) horn
grey matter
white matter
lateral horn
meninges
pia mater
arachnoid
dura mater
anterior (ventral) horn
cell bodies of motor neurones
subdural space
anterior (ventral) root

Diagram of General Plan of Spinal Cord

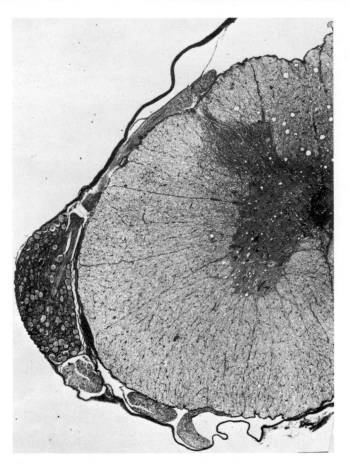

110. **Spinal cord,** roots and ganglion, T.S. (rabbit), mag. 15 ×

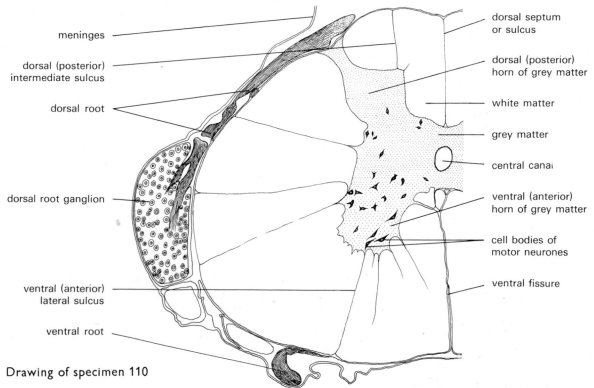

meninges

dorsal (posterior)
intermediate sulcus

dorsal root

dorsal root ganglion

ventral (anterior)
lateral sulcus

ventral root

dorsal septum
or sulcus

dorsal (posterior)
horn of grey matter

white matter

grey matter

central canal

ventral (anterior)
horn of grey matter

cell bodies of
motor neurones

ventral fissure

Drawing of specimen 110

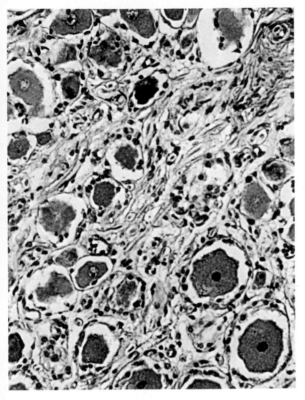

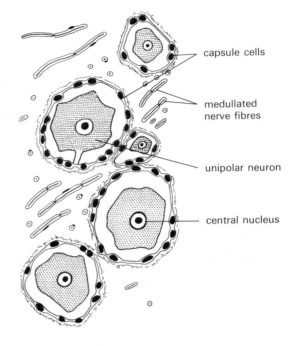

capsule cells

medullated
nerve fibres

unipolar neuron

central nucleus

111. **Dorsal root ganglion**, L.S. (baboon), mag. 350×

Drawing of specimen 111

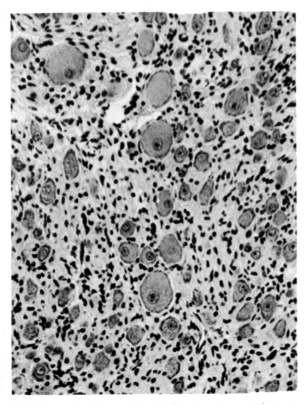

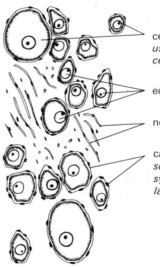

cell bodies of neurons
*usually smaller than the nerve
cells of dorsal root ganglion*

eccentric nuclei

non-medullated nerve fibres

capsule cells
*some of the nerve cells in
sympathetic ganglia
lack capsules*

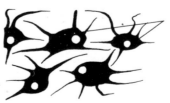

multipolar neurons –
with irregular shape

**Drawing of nerve cells from
a silver-stained preparation**

112. **Sympathetic ganglion**, L.S. (baboon), mag. 250×

Drawing of specimen 112

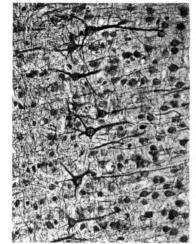

114. **Cerebrum**, pyramidal cells, L.S. (monkey), mag. 400 ×

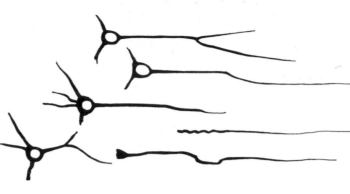

Diagram of pyramidal cells

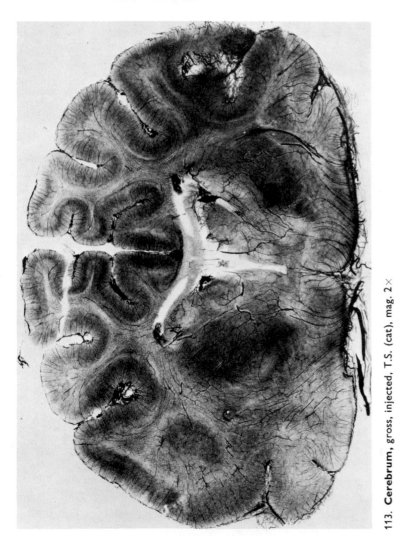

113. **Cerebrum**, gross, injected, T.S. (cat), mag. 2 ×

grey matter of cerebral cortex
white matter
convolutions of cortex
blood vessels of the grey matter
receive blood from carotid artery
lateral ventricle
corpus callosum
third ventricle
internal capsule
blood vessels in the pia mater
thalamus
lentiform nucleus
blood vessels of the white matter
these are relatively sparse

Drawing of specimen 113

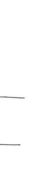

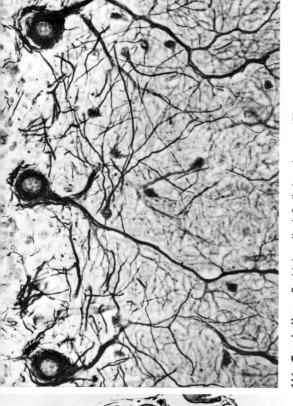

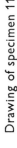

116. **Cerebellum,** Purkinje cells, L.S. (baboon), mag. 450 ×

bipolar granule cell
entry-route for impulses
granular layer
axon of Purkinje cell
Purkinje cell layer
basket of fibrils
surrounding Purkinje cell
branching dendrites
of Purkinje cell
molecular layer
basket cells
*each basket cell picks
up impulses from
granule cell axons and
passes them to several
Purkinje cells via
baskets of fibres*

Drawing of specimen 116

115. **Cerebellum,** gross, L.S. (baboon), mag. 6 ×

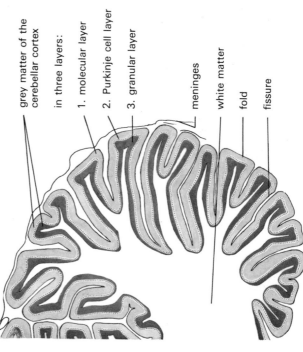

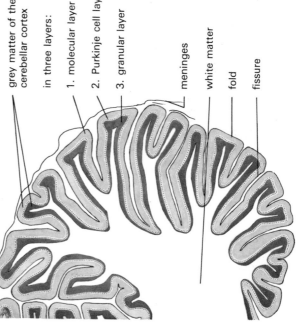

grey matter of the
cerebellar cortex

in three layers:

1. molecular layer
2. Purkinje cell layer
3. granular layer

meninges
white matter
fold
fissure

Drawing of specimen 115

133

THE ENDOCRINE SYSTEM

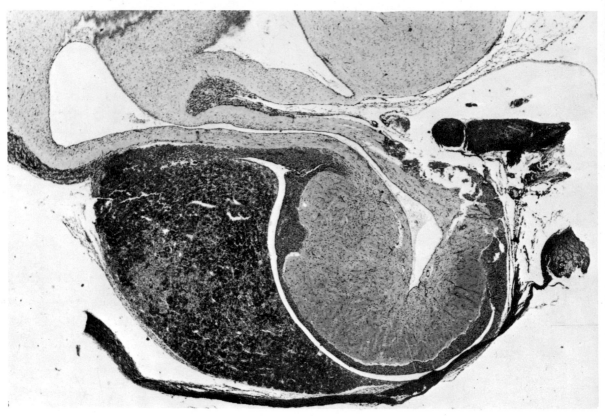

117. **Pituitary gland,** L.S. (cat), mag. 32×

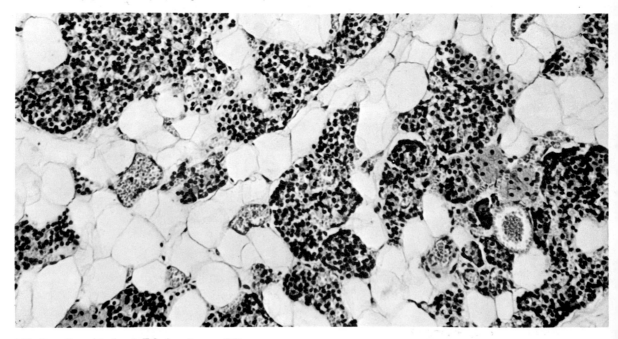

118. **Parathyroid gland,** T.S. (man), mag. 350×

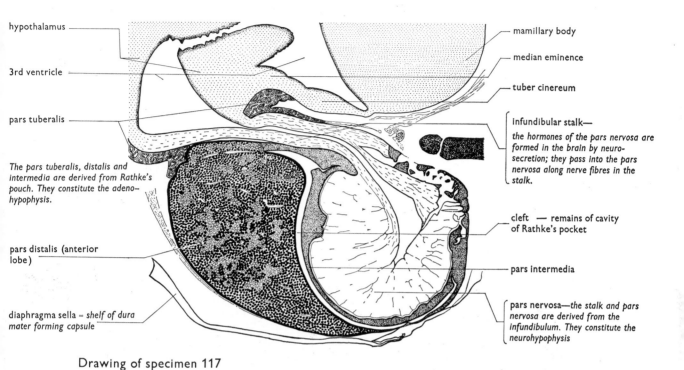

hypothalamus

3rd ventricle

pars tuberalis

The pars tuberalis, distalis and intermedia are derived from Rathke's pouch. They constitute the adeno–hypophysis.

pars distalis (anterior lobe)

diaphragma sella = *shelf of dura mater forming capsule*

mamillary body

median eminence

tuber cinereum

infundibular stalk—
the hormones of the pars nervosa are formed in the brain by neuro-secretion; they pass into the pars nervosa along nerve fibres in the stalk.

cleft — *remains of cavity of Rathke's pocket*

pars intermedia

pars nervosa—*the stalk and pars nervosa are derived from the infundibulum. They constitute the neurohypophysis*

Drawing of specimen 117

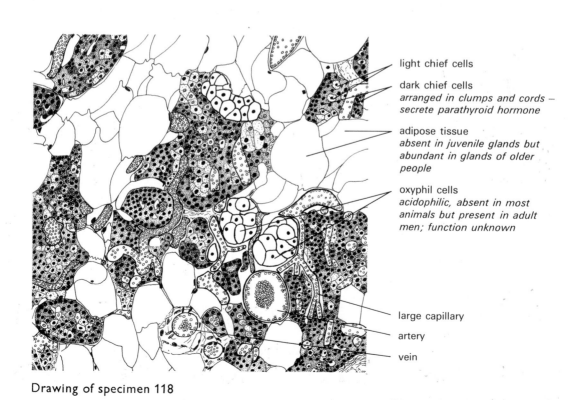

light chief cells

dark chief cells
arranged in clumps and cords – secrete parathyroid hormone

adipose tissue
absent in juvenile glands but abundant in glands of older people

oxyphil cells
acidophilic, absent in most animals but present in adult men; function unknown

large capillary

artery

vein

Drawing of specimen 118

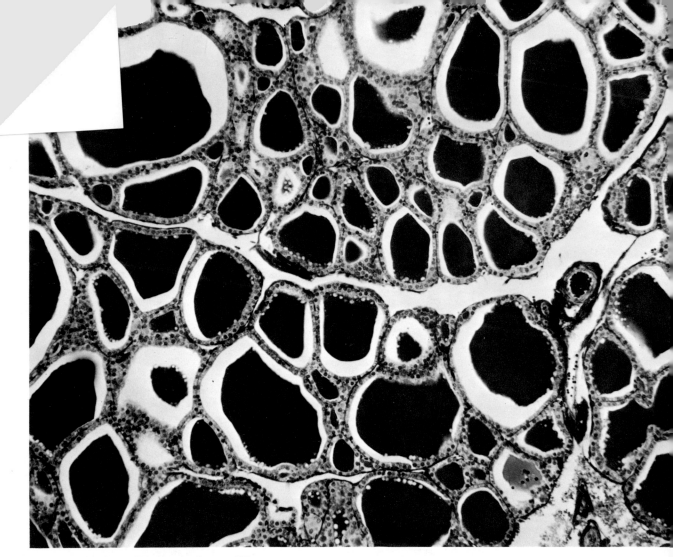

119. **Thyroid gland,** T.S. (monkey), mag. 350×

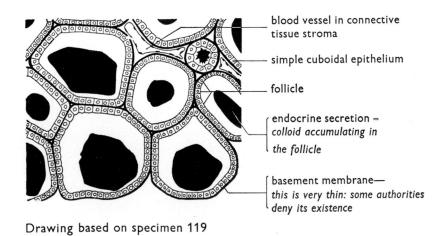

— blood vessel in connective tissue stroma

— simple cuboidal epithelium

— follicle

{ endocrine secretion = *colloid accumulating in the follicle*

{ basement membrane— *this is very thin: some authorities deny its existence*

Drawing based on specimen 119

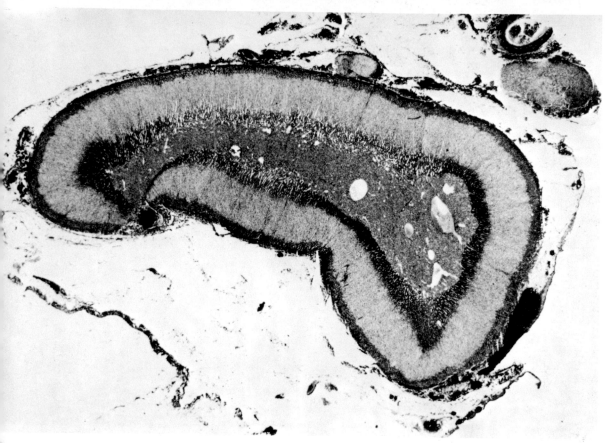

. **Adrenal gland gross,** T.S. (monkey), mag. 15×

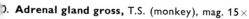

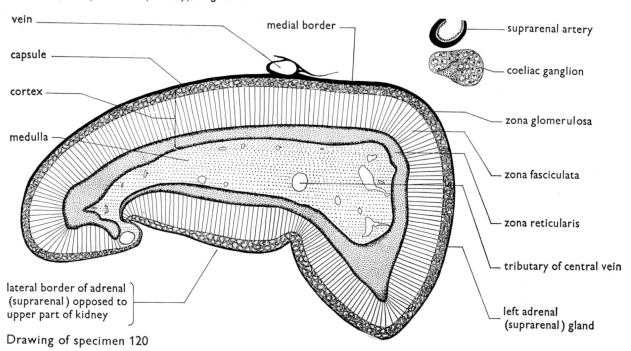

vein

capsule

cortex

medulla

medial border

suprarenal artery

coeliac ganglion

zona glomerulosa

zona fasciculata

zona reticularis

tributary of central vein

left adrenal
(suprarenal) gland

lateral border of adrenal
(suprarenal) opposed to
upper part of kidney

Drawing of specimen 120

137

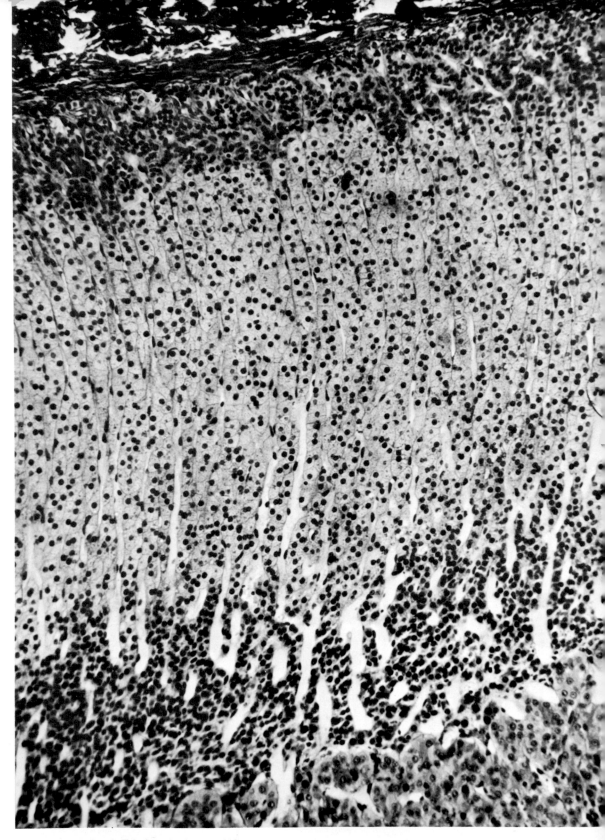

121. **Adrenal gland,** T.S. (monkey), mag. 110×

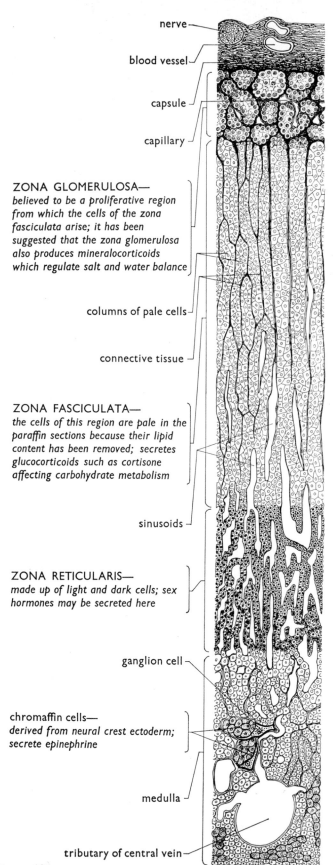

nerve

blood vessel

capsule

capillary

ZONA GLOMERULOSA—
*believed to be a proliferative region
from which the cells of the zona
fasciculata arise; it has been
suggested that the zona glomerulosa
also produces mineralocorticoids
which regulate salt and water balance*

columns of pale cells

connective tissue

ZONA FASCICULATA—
*the cells of this region are pale in the
paraffin sections because their lipid
content has been removed; secretes
glucocorticoids such as cortisone
affecting carbohydrate metabolism*

sinusoids

ZONA RETICULARIS—
*made up of light and dark cells; sex
hormones may be secreted here*

ganglion cell

chromaffin cells—
*derived from neural crest ectoderm;
secrete epinephrine*

medulla

tributary of central vein

Drawing of specimen 121

THE CIRCULATORY SYSTEM

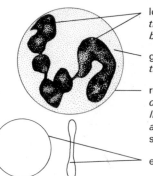

lobed nucleus
*the number of lobes varies
between 2 and 5*

granules in cytoplasm –
these are lysosomes

round shape
*only in fixed specimens:
living neutrophils are
amoeboid
size 10–15μ*

erythrocyte – for comparison

Drawing of specimen 122

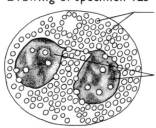

ingested bacteria
*bacteria ingested by
phagocytosis are destroyed
by the proteolytic
enzymes of lysosomes*

nucleus

erythrocyte

Drawing of specimen 123

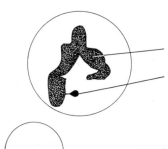

lobed nucleus

drumstick
*this is an X chromosome
seen in about 5% of the
neutrophils in blood
smears of female blood*

erythrocyte

Drawing of specimen 124

eosinophilic granules
*these are larger than those
of neutrophils, and stain
orange with eosin*

bilobed nucleus
*eosinophils also ingest
bacteria, but to a lesser
extent than neutrophils*

size 10–15μ

erythrocyte

Drawing of specimen 125

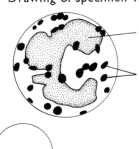

lobed nucleus
*not all basophils have
lobed nuclei*

granules
*contain heparin, histamine,
and serotonin; cells with
few granules have recently
discharged their contents
size 10–15μ*

erythrocyte

Drawing of specimen 126

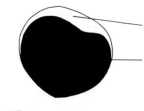

cytoplasm
stain deep blue

nucleus

*size 10–11μ
lymphocytes are mobile an
can escape through capilla
walls into the tissues;
they produce antibodies*

erythrocyte

Drawing of specimen 127

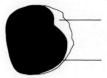

cytoplasm
stain deep blue

nucleus

size 8–9μ

erythrocyte

140   **Drawing of specimen 128**

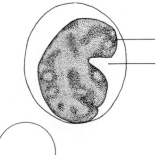

indented nucleus

cytoplasm
*stains pale blue, contains
lysosomes
size 18–20μ
monocytes, which ingest
bacteria, are the largest
blood cells*

erythrocyte

Drawing of specimen 129

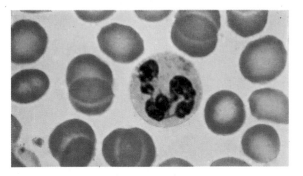

122. Neutrophil

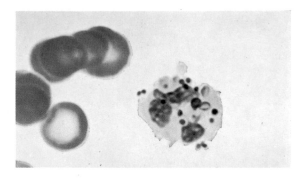

123. Phagocytosis

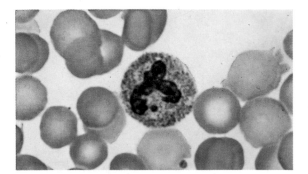

124. Neutrophil, with drumstick

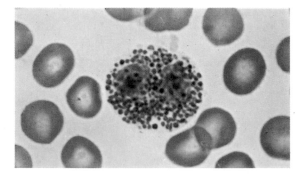

125. Eosinophil

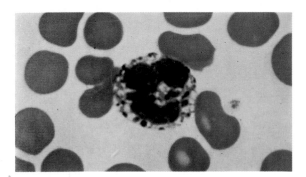

126. Basophil

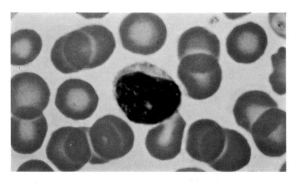

127. Large lymphocyte

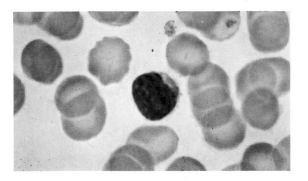

128. Small lymphocyte

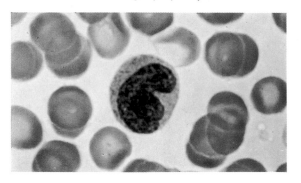

129. Monocyte

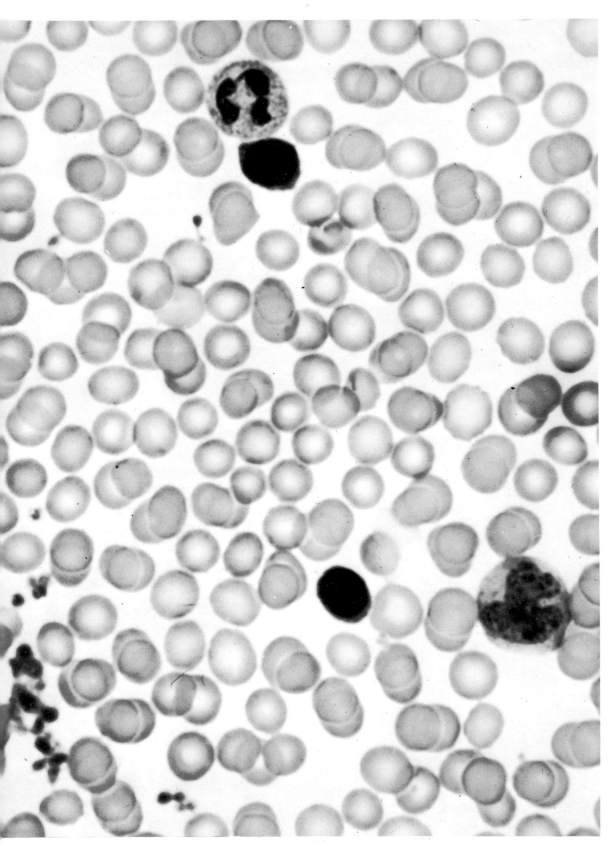

130. **Blood film** (man), mag. 1600 $\times$

Peripheral blood culture technique for chromosome preparations

Some human diseases are caused by abnormalities in the number and morphology of the chromosomes and it is therefore essential for diagnostic purposes to be able to examine the chromosomes. Chromosomes can be seen as distinct bodies in the metaphase plate of a dividing nucleus, but suitable examples of this stage are rare in normal tissues. This problem can be overcome by stimulating cell division. When leucocytes from a blood sample are stimulated with phytohaemagglutinin and then grown in tissue culture medium, they reach an actively dividing phase in three days. Mitosis is arrested at metaphase by adding colchicine which inhibits centromere division and spindle formation. Mitosis is halted but the unseparated chromatids continue to coil; a delay of two hours before the cells are harvested produces chromosomes that are shorter and more distinct than normal. The harvested leucocytes are placed in a hypotonic solution in order to make them swell and allow the chromosomes on the metaphase plate to spread out and separate from each other. The swollen cells are fixed in acetic-methanol, air dried on a slide and stained with acetic-orcein. Specimen 131 illustrates this technique. The chromosome number for an individual is determined by counting twenty or more plates, the normal number being 46. The morphology of the chromosomes is studied from the preparation and from an enlarged photomicrograph of a good spread. The latter is cut up and the chromosomes arranged in pairs according to size and position of the centromeres; specimen 132 is an orderly arrangement, or karyotype, of the spread chromosomes in 131. The pairs of autosomes in a karyotype are serially numbered from 1 to 22 in decreasing order of size; the pair of sex chromosomes is designated XX in females and XY in males. The arrangement of chromosomes into the groups A to G is based on such criteria as the position of the centromere and the ratio of arm lengths. The X chromosomes closely resemble members of group C, and the Y chromosome is placed in group G. An individual chromosome can be placed in its appropriate group more readily than it can be allocated a serial number. Folds may make chromosomes appear to be shorter than they are, e.g. one of group C in 132.

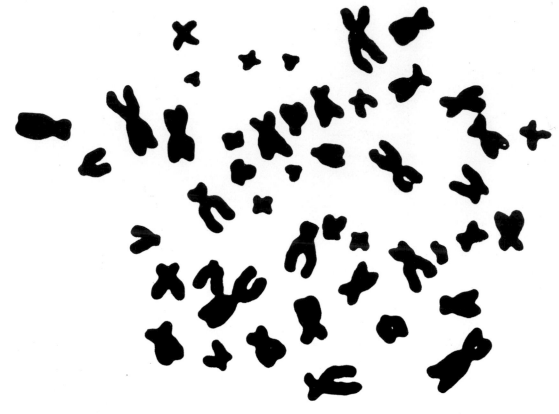

131. **Chromosome spread,** metaphase plate (man), mag. 4000 ×

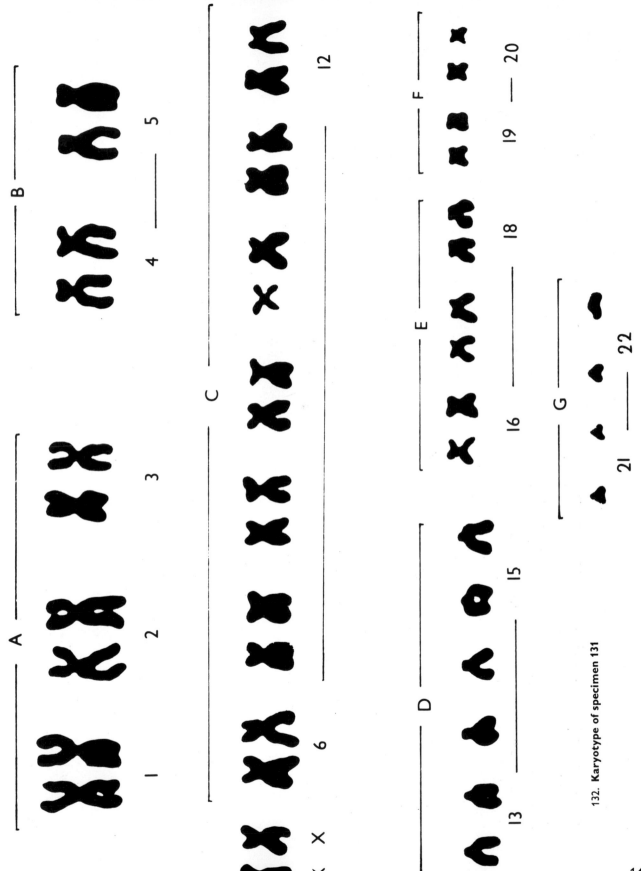

132. Karyotype of specimen 131

143

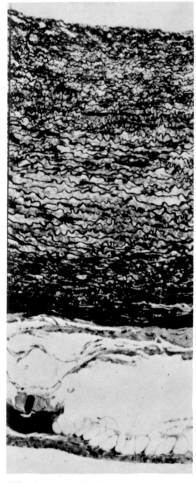

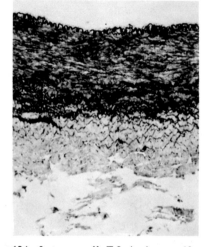

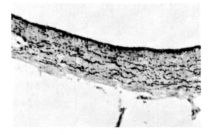

133. Aorta wall, T.S. (cat), mag. 60×   **134. Artery wall,** T.S. (cat), mag. 60×   **135. Vein wall,** T.S. (cat), mag. 60×

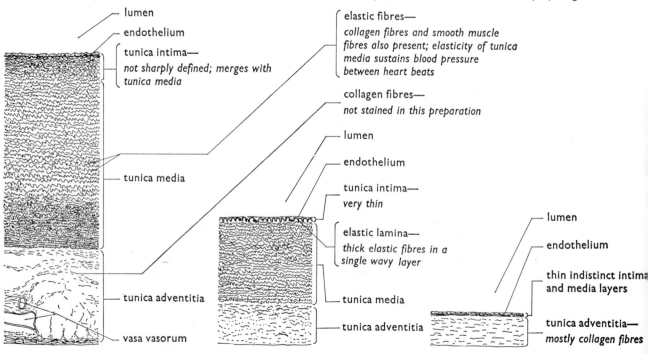

lumen

endothelium

tunica intima—
not sharply defined; merges with tunica media

tunica media

tunica adventitia

vasa vasorum

elastic fibres—
collagen fibres and smooth muscle fibres also present; elasticity of tunica media sustains blood pressure between heart beats

collagen fibres—
not stained in this preparation

lumen

endothelium

tunica intima—
very thin

elastic lamina—
thick elastic fibres in a single wavy layer

tunica media

tunica adventitia

lumen

endothelium

thin indistinct intima and media layers

tunica adventitia—
mostly collagen fibres

144   Drawing of specimen 133   Drawing of specimen 134   Drawing of specimen 135

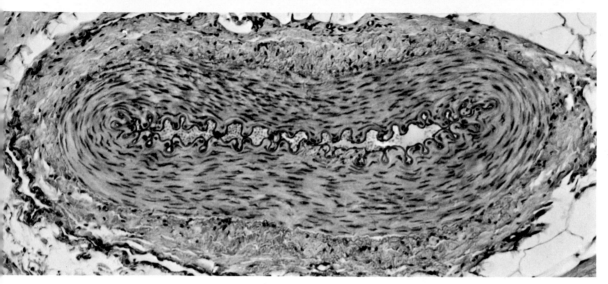

36. Muscular artery wall, T.S. (man), mag. 60×

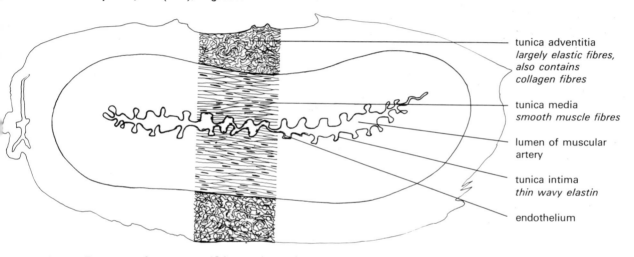

tunica adventitia
*largely elastic fibres,
also contains
collagen fibres*

tunica media
smooth muscle fibres

lumen of muscular
artery

tunica intima
thin wavy elastin

endothelium

Drawing of specimen 136

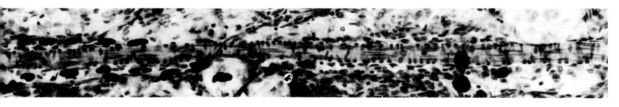

37. Arteriole (mammal), mag. 300×

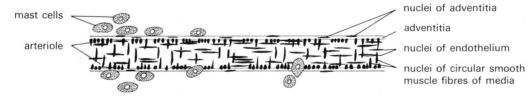

mast cells

arteriole

nuclei of adventitia

adventitia

nuclei of endothelium

nuclei of circular smooth
muscle fibres of media

Drawing of specimen 137

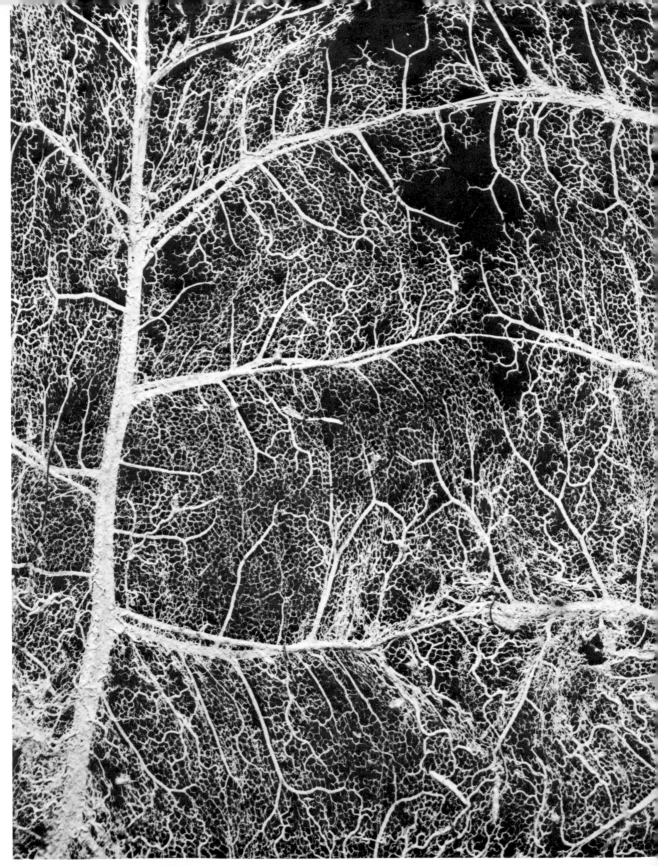

138. **Capillaries,** injected (rat ileum stretch), mag. 50 ×

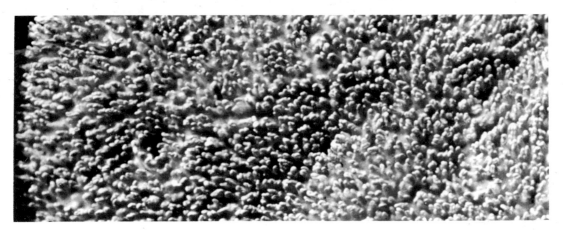

139. **Capillaries,** injected, surface loops (human finger pad), mag. 75×

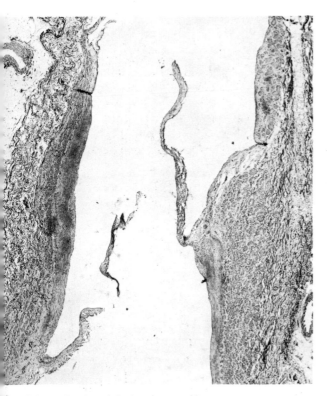

140. **Vein and valve,** L.S. (man), mag. 11×

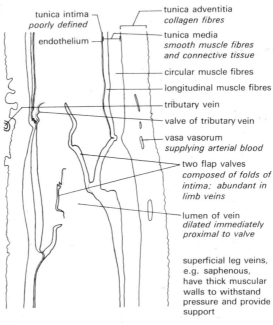

Drawing of specimen 140

tunica intima
poorly defined

endothelium

tunica adventitia
collagen fibres

tunica media
*smooth muscle fibres
and connective tissue*

circular muscle fibres

longitudinal muscle fibres

tributary vein

valve of tributary vein

vasa vasorum
supplying arterial blood

two flap valves
*composed of folds of
intima; abundant in
limb veins*

lumen of vein
*dilated immediately
proximal to valve*

superficial leg veins,
e.g. saphenous,
have thick muscular
walls to withstand
pressure and provide
support

MAIN FEATURES OF THE VASCULAR SYSTEM

TYPE OF VESSEL	TUNICA INTIMA	TUNICA MEDIA	TUNICA ADVENTITIA
ELASTIC ARTERIES (large, conducting arteries, e.g. aorta).	Forms a fifth of total thickness of wall; composed of loose connective tissue containing less elastin than media; inner surface lined with a simple squamous endothelium resting on a basement membrane; the internal elastic lamina marks the outer boundary.	Forms the major part of wall; composed of concentrically arranged laminae of elastin in an amorphous ground substance with fine elastic fibres, collagen fibres and smooth muscle fibres between laminae; the smooth muscle fibre cells of all blood vessels are of a special kind which produces ground substance, elastin and collagen.	A thin layer composed of elastic and collagen fibres; the adventitia merges with the surrounding connective tissue; contains small blood vessels, the vasa vasorum, which enter the outer layers of the tunica media.
MUSCULAR ARTERIES (small distributing arteries, e.g. inferior intestinal artery).	A thin layer lined by an endothelium and bounded by internal elastic lamina; the wavy appearance of endothelium due to contraction of wall after death; subendothelial layer composed of a few undifferentiated smooth muscle cells in loose connective tissue.	A thick layer composed of circularly arranged smooth muscle fibres held together by elastic fibres in larger arteries and by a mixture of elastic and collagen fibres in smaller distributing arteries.	The thickness of this layer is a half to two-thirds that of the tunica media; largely composed of elastic fibres; collagen also present in larger distributing arteries; have vasa vasorum.
ARTERIOLES	A thin layer with endothelium resting on internal elastic lamina; intima reduced to endothelium in smallest arterioles.	Consists of a single layer of exceptionally short smooth muscle fibres circularly arranged which regulate flow through capillaries.	Of the same thickness as the media; composed of collagen and elastic fibres in larger arterioles and collagen in smallest arterioles and very thin.
CAPILLARIES	Endothelium consists of simple squamous epithelium resting on a basement membrane; EMs show pinocytotic vesicles in the endothelium, and reveal that some visceral capillaries are fenestrated; non-contractile pericytes are scattered on outside of endothelium where they secrete basement membrane and act as phagocytes.	Absent.	Absent.
SINUSOIDS	A continuous endothelium is absent and walls consist of scattered cells some being phagocytic.	Absent.	Absent.
VENULES	A continuous endothelium is present with abundant pericytes; support provided by collagen fibres.	Absent.	Absent.
SMALL AND MEDIUM VEINS (e.g. inferior mesenteric vein).	Endothelium present but rest of intima poorly defined; folds of intima form flap valves in veins of extremities.	A thinner layer than the tunica media of companion artery; circular smooth muscle fibres more irregularly arranged than in companion artery.	This is the thickest of the three layers; composed of collagen fibres.
SUPERFICIAL VEINS (e.g. saphenous vein).	Endothelium present but rest of intima poorly defined; folds strengthened by elastic fibres form flap valves.	This is a thick layer which has to withstand the hydrostatic pressure of a long column of blood unaided by the support of surrounding tissue; composed of an inner layer of longitudinal and an outer layer of circular smooth muscle bounded by elastic fibres.	Also a thick layer supplied with vasa vasorum.
LARGE VEINS (e.g. vena cava).	Endothelium present but rest of intima poorly developed.	Poorly developed with little smooth muscle.	A thick coat containing collagen and elastic fibres; may contain longitudinal smooth muscle fibres.

THE MAIN FEATURES OF THE LYMPHATIC SYSTEM (salient features in bold print)

LYMPHATIC ORGAN	CAPSULE	HILUS	EPITHELIUM	CORTEX	MEDULLA	LYMPHATIC NODULES (= FOLLICLES)	LYMPHATIC VESSELS	SINUSES
LYMPH NODE	Composed of fibrous connective tissue with trabeculae projecting into node; **adipose tissue** on outer surface of capsule; **subcapsular sinus** beneath capsule.	Present.	Absent; lymph nodes develop from mesenchyme cells.	**Present** in varying amounts; conspicuous when medulla is poorly developed; composed of diffuse tissue **containing lymphatic nodules.**	**Present** in varying amounts; conspicuous when cortex is poorly developed; composed of **medullary cords** with **lymphatic sinuses** between cords; **cords contain plasma cells.**	**Present in the cortex;** nodules have 'germinal' centres.	Afferent vessels enter convex surface of node, efferent vessels leave from the hilus.	**Lymphatic sinuses** present in medulla and beneath capsule; **lymph nodes filter lymph.**
SPLEEN	Composed of fibrous connective tissue with trabeculae containing larger veins; no adipose tissue.	Present close to medial border.	Absent; spleen develops from mesenchyme cells.	Absent.	Absent.	**Present in white pulp;** nodules may have 'germinal' centres; **white pulp is distributed along small arteries.**	Absent.	**Venous sinuses** present in **red pulp; spleen filters blood.**
THYMUS	Composed of a **thin layer** of connective tissue extending into **and dividing thymus into lobules.**	Absent.	Absent; thymus develops from mesenchyme cells.	Present; has a **darkly stained appearance.**	Present; stains pale; **contains Hassall's corpuscles.**	Absent.	Absent apart from some in capsule.	Absent.
LINGUAL TONSIL	Absent.	Absent.	**A stratified non-keratinized squamous epithelium** extends into tonsil to **form crypts; ducts of underlying mucous glands open into crypts and flush them out.**	Absent.	Absent.	**Present clustered round crypts;** nodules have 'germinal' centres surrounded by closely packed small lymphocytes.	Present.	Absent.
PALATINE TONSIL	**Present on deep aspect;** composed of fibrous connective tissue.	Absent.	**A stratified non-keratinized squamous epithelium** extends into tonsil to form **primary crypts** from which arise **secondary crypts; crypts not flushed out** by mucous gland ducts and **debris tends to collect in 'tonsils'** which may have to be removed.	Absent.	Absent.	Present in loose lymphatic tissue; 'germinal' centres may or may not be present; **nodules usually in a single layer** around crypts and below epithelium.	Present.	Absent.
PHARYNGEAL TONSIL	**Present but less well defined** than in palatine tonsil.	Absent.	**A pseudo-stratified columnar epithelium** extends into tonsil as **folds and not as crypts; may obstruct air passage** which lymphoid tissue becomes enlarged and 'adenoids' have to be removed.	Absent.	Absent.	Present in loose lymphatic tissue; **more diffuse** than in laryngeal and palatine tonsil.	Present.	Absent.
PEYER'S PATCHES	**Absent.**	Absent.	Related to **simple columnar epithelium of ileum.**	Absent.	Absent.	Present as **isolated or confluent nodules in** ilium on opposite side **to the mesentery;** active 'germinal' centres present; smaller lymphoid aggregates occur in other parts of the alimentary canal.	Present, draining to regional lymph nodes.	Absent.

THE LYMPHATIC SYSTEM

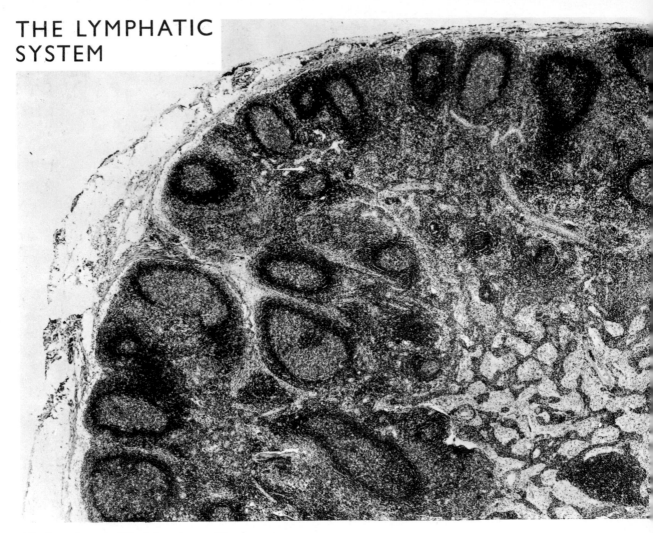

141. **Lymph node**, T.S. (baboon), mag. 20×

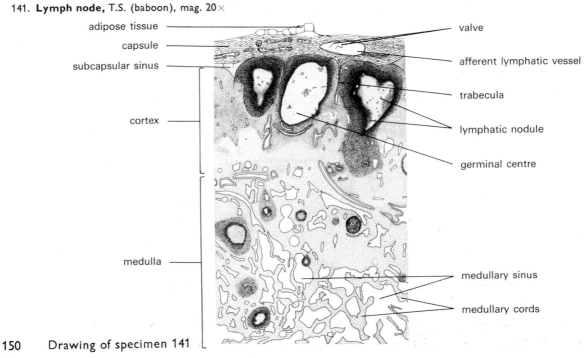

adipose tissue

capsule

subcapsular sinus

cortex

medulla

valve

afferent lymphatic vessel

trabecula

lymphatic nodule

germinal centre

medullary sinus

medullary cords

Drawing of specimen 141

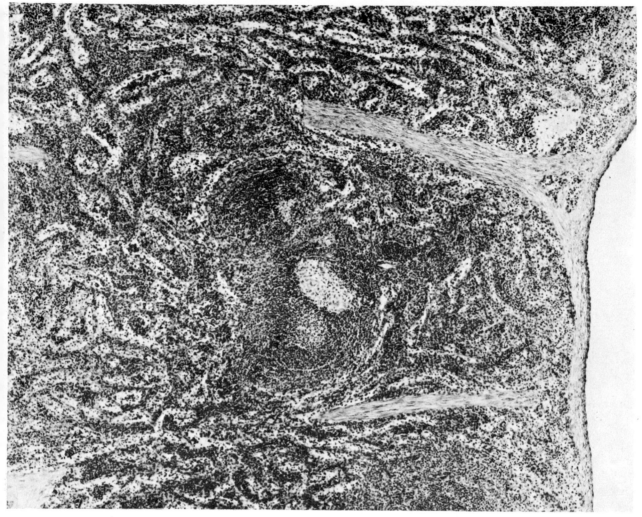

142. **Spleen,** T.S. (man), mag. 35×

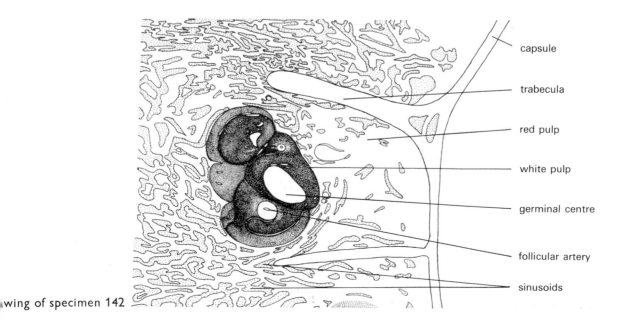

capsule

trabecula

red pulp

white pulp

germinal centre

follicular artery

sinusoids

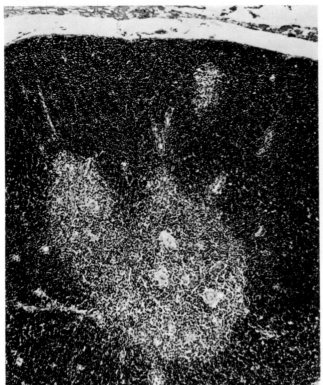

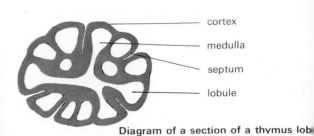

cortex

medulla

septum

lobule

Diagram of a section of a thymus lob

connective tissue capsule
this extends into the thym
to form septa dividing eac
lobe into lobules

cortex
heavily infiltrated with
lymphocytes

medulla
contains fewer lymphocyt

blood vessel

Hassall's corpuscle
rings of flattened epithelia
cells surrounding dead
material — found only in
the thymus

Drawing of specimen 143

143. Thymus, T.S. (mammal), mag. 30×

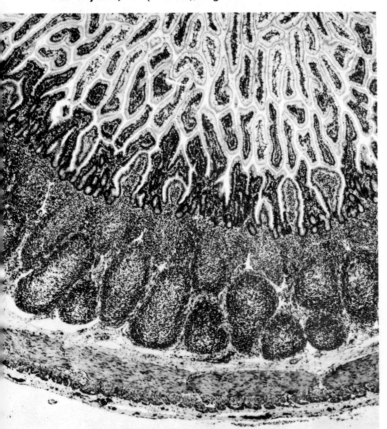

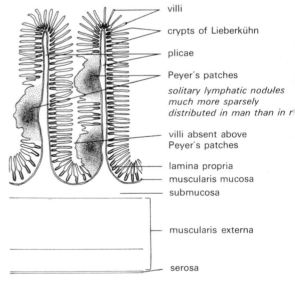

villi

crypts of Lieberkühn

plicae

Peyer's patches
solitary lymphatic nodules
much more sparsely
distributed in man than in r

villi absent above
Peyer's patches

lamina propria
muscularis mucosa

submucosa

muscularis externa

serosa

Drawing of Peyer's patches in human jejunum

144. Peyer's patches, T.S. (rat), mag. 35×

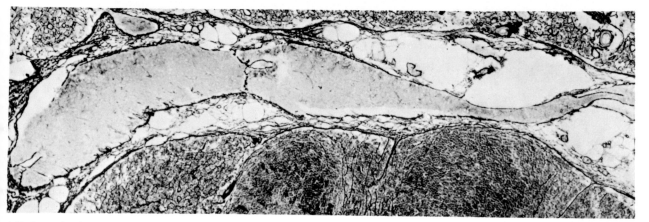

145. Lymphatic vessel and valves, L.S. (mammal), mag. 65×

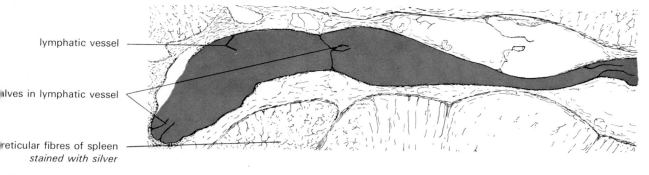

lymphatic vessel —

valves in lymphatic vessel —

reticular fibres of spleen —
stained with silver

Drawing of specimen 145

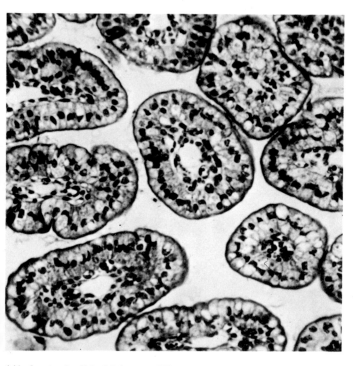

146. Lacteals, T.S. (pig), mag. 350×

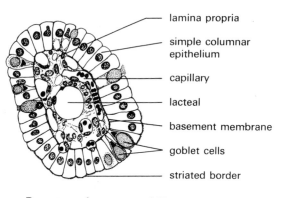

lamina propria

simple columnar
epithelium

capillary

lacteal

basement membrane

goblet cells

striated border

Drawing of specimen 146

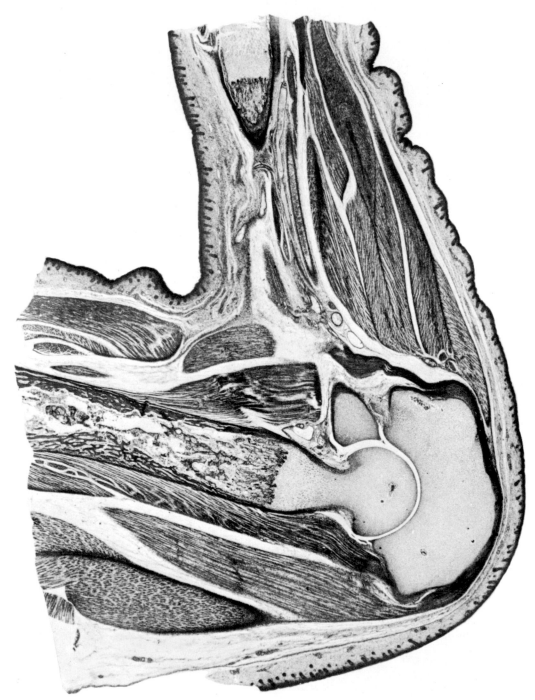

147. **Elbow joint**, L.S. (rat), mag. 12×

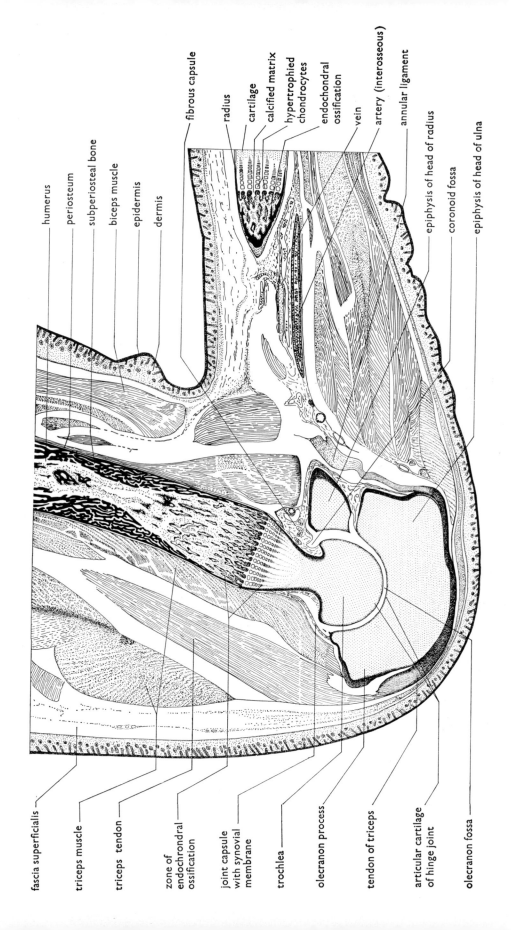

humerus

periosteum

subperiosteal bone

biceps muscle

epidermis

dermis

fibrous capsule

radius

cartilage

calcified matrix

hypertrophied chondrocytes

endochondral ossification

vein

artery (interosseous)

annular ligament

epiphysis of head of radius

coronoid fossa

epiphysis of head of ulna

fascia superficialis

triceps muscle

triceps tendon

zone of endochrondral ossification

joint capsule with synovial membrane

trochlea

olecranon process

tendon of triceps

articular cartilage of hinge joint

olecranon fossa

Drawing of specimen 147

155

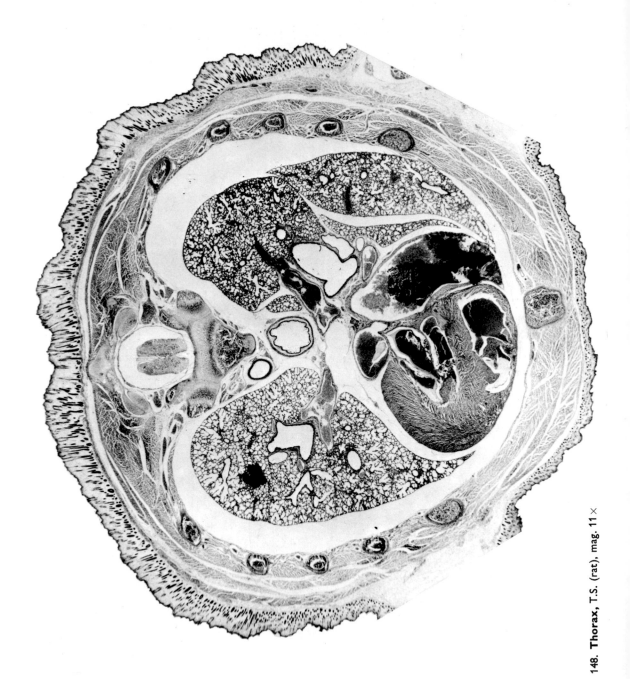

148. **Thorax**, T.S. (rat), mag. 11 ×

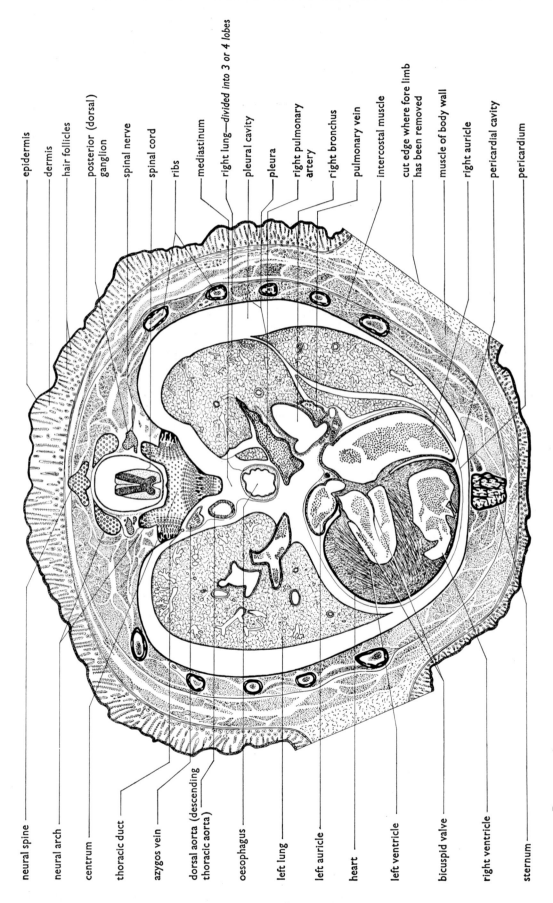

epidermis

dermis

hair follicles

posterior (dorsal) ganglion

spinal nerve

spinal cord

ribs

mediastinum

right lung—*divided into 3 or 4 lobes*

pleural cavity

pleura

right pulmonary artery

right bronchus

pulmonary vein

intercostal muscle

cut edge where fore limb has been removed

muscle of body wall

right auricle

pericardial cavity

pericardium

neural spine

neural arch

centrum

thoracic duct

azygos vein

dorsal aorta (descending thoracic aorta)

oesophagus

left lung

left auricle

heart

left ventricle

bicuspid valve

right ventricle

sternum

Drawing of specimen 148

157

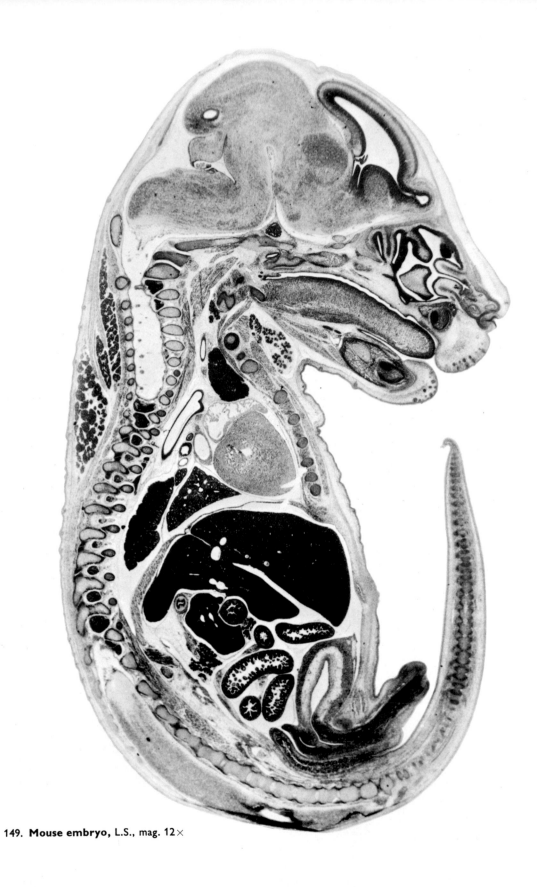

149. **Mouse embryo**, L.S., mag. 12×

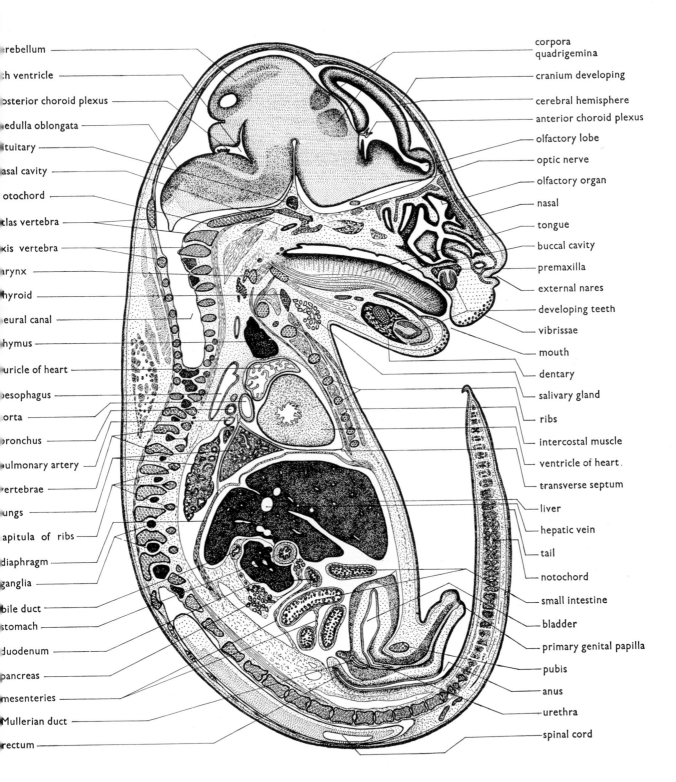

cerebellum
4th ventricle
posterior choroid plexus
medulla oblongata
pituitary
nasal cavity
notochord
atlas vertebra
axis vertebra
larynx
thyroid
neural canal
thymus
auricle of heart
oesophagus
aorta
bronchus
pulmonary artery
vertebrae
lungs
capitula of ribs
diaphragm
ganglia
bile duct
stomach
duodenum
pancreas
mesenteries
Mullerian duct
rectum

corpora quadrigemina
cranium developing
cerebral hemisphere
anterior choroid plexus
olfactory lobe
optic nerve
olfactory organ
nasal
tongue
buccal cavity
premaxilla
external nares
developing teeth
vibrissae
mouth
dentary
salivary gland
ribs
intercostal muscle
ventricle of heart
transverse septum
liver
hepatic vein
tail
notochord
small intestine
bladder
primary genital papilla
pubis
anus
urethra
spinal cord

Drawing of specimen 149

159